Plant-Based Diet

The Essential Cookbook to Lose Weight, Live Longer, and Be Healthier with Delicious Plant-Based Recipes - Includes 4-Week Meal Prep Plan (Beginners Friendly)

Michelle Thomasson

© **Copyright 2019 - All rights reserved.**

The content contained within this book may not be reproduced, duplicated or transmitted without direct written permission from the author or the publisher.

Under no circumstances will any blame or legal responsibility be held against the publisher, or author, for any damages, reparation, or monetary loss due to the information contained within this book, either directly or indirectly.

Legal Notice:

This book is copyright protected. It is only for personal use. You cannot amend, distribute, sell, use, quote or paraphrase any part, or the content within this book, without the consent of the author or publisher.

Disclaimer Notice:

Please note the information contained within this document is for educational and entertainment purposes only. All effort has been executed to present accurate, up to date, reliable, complete information. No warranties of any kind are declared or implied. Readers acknowledge that the author is not engaging in the rendering of legal, financial, medical or professional advice. The content within this book has been derived from various sources. Please consult a licensed professional before attempting any techniques outlined in this book.

By reading this document, the reader agrees that under no circumstances is the author responsible for any losses, direct or indirect, that are incurred as a result of the use of information contained within this document, including, but not limited to, errors, omissions, or inaccuracies.

Table of Contents

Introduction

Chapter 1: What Does "Plant-Based" Mean?

   Vegetarian, Vegan, and Plant-Based: What Are the Differences?

      What about Veganism?

      Nutrition and Misconceptions

Chapter 2: Plants and Your Health

Chapter 3: Transitioning to a Plant-Based Diet

   How to Calculate Your Caloric Needs

Chapter 4: Plant-Based Foods: A Guide

   What to Add to My Shopping List

Chapter 5: Recipes

   Smoothies and Breakfast

      Mocha Smoothie

      Mint Choc-Chip Smoothie

      Blueberry Smoothie

      Cinnamon Smoothie

      Creamy Orange Smoothie

- Peanut Butter Smoothie
- Berry Smoothie
- Pumpkin Breakfast Cookies
- Pancakes
- Chickpea and Onion Omelet
- Gingerbread Waffles
- Breakfast Grits Bowl
- Tofu Scramble
- Vegan Crepes
- Fig Oatmeal Breakfast Bake
- Vegan French Toast

Soups
- Spicy Squash Soup
- Tomato Soup
- Mushroom Soup
- Noodle Soup

Salads and Sides
- Cinnamon-Apple Bread
- Zucchini Bread
- Tortilla Roll-Ups

Coconut Potatoes

Grilled Butternut Squash

Chili

Avo and Noodle Salad

Fig and Arugula Salad

Spring Salad

Summer Salad

Chickpea Meatballs and Romaine Salad

Roasted Summer Veggies

Roasted Cauli-Wedges

Roasted Pumpkin and Brussels Sprouts

Sun-Dried Tomato Quiche

Main Dishes

Sloppy Joe

Zucchini Lasagna

Crispy Tofu Stir-Fry

Mac and Cheese

Avo-Kale-Veggie Bowl

Mushroom-Asparagus Bowl

Veggie Bolognese

Sweet Potato and Lentil Curry

Orange-Tofu Stir-Fry

Lentil-Tahini Burger

Chickpea and Bulgur Wheat Burgers

Black Bean and Mushroom Burger

Mushroom and Zucchini Bowl

Butternut Chickpea Stew

Cauli-Korma

Snacks and Appetizers

    Chocolate Chip Granola Bars

    Sandwiches with Hummus Spread

    Coconut Bacon

    Black Bean Tostada

Desserts

    Ginger Cookies

    Choc-Mint Ice Cream

    Spicy Chocolate Fudge

    Basic Vanilla Buttercream Frosting

    Chocolate Frosting

    Chocolate Cupcakes

- Cinnamon Rolls
- Peppermint Strawberry Cheesecake
- Sugar Cookies

Basic Sauces and Condiments
- Cream Sauce
- Kale-and-Walnut Pesto
- Spicy Vegan Dip
- Vegan Ranch 1
- Vegan Ranch 2
- BBQ Tahini
- Vegan Sour Cream
- Cheese Dip
- Thai Peanut Sauce
- Salad Dressing
- Vegan Alfredo Sauce
- Hummus
- Walnut Butter
- Cashew Butter
- Roasted Almond Butter
- Tomato-Basil Sauce

    Vegan Parmesan

    Chimichurri

  Drinks

    Strawberry Milk

    Apple Cider

    Hot Christmas Rum

Chapter 6: The Plant-Based Meal Plan

  Week 1

  Week 2

  Week 3

  Week 4

Conclusion

Bibliography

Introduction

There is a lot of controversy around the idea of following a plant-based diet. Is it just as a means to eat healthier, or is it a way to limit the impact you have on the environment (think vegan)?

There are several considerations when switching to any new diet, and a lot of research is often required. What works for one person would not necessarily work for another. However, adding in extra nutrient-rich vegetables to your diet will certainly benefit you, regardless of your choice to keep including animal-based protein.

This book contains all the information you will need to make the transition to a plant-based diet, including a four-week meal plan with accompanying healthy recipes that are easy to follow and taste fantastic.

Chapter 1: What Does "Plant-Based" Mean?

There are a lot of conflicting ideas regarding the extent a person can be plant-based and still eat meat. That being said, the general consensus is that following a plant-based diet is one where the main focus lies in your plant-based proteins as well as a variety of vegetables, aiming to reduce or eliminate the intake of meat products as a whole.

"Plant-based" would simply be seen as shifting the main focus of your meals, having vegetables make up 80–90% of your plate and the remainder a meat-based protein. While many believe that to be plant-based means you need to be fully vegan for that to apply, it is not necessarily the case.

Vegetarian, Vegan, and Plant-Based: What Are the Differences?

Vegetarian diets have been around as long as anyone can remember. There are variations in this type of eating due to various reasons, ranging from religion to dietary requirements.

The person's intake of animal-based proteins is dependent on the type of vegetarian diet they have chosen. While those who consume these animal-based proteins or by-products are not wholly considered to be true vegetarians, they do still, technically, fall under the same category:

1. **Lacto-ovo vegetarians** avoid all animal-based proteins with the exception of dairy and eggs. Therefore, they consume items such as cheese and mayonnaise.

2. **Lacto vegetarians** avoid all animal-based proteins as well as eggs but with the exception of dairy products, such as yogurt and milk.

3. **Ovo vegetarians** avoid all animal-based proteins as well as dairy products but with the exception of eggs.

4. **Pescatarians** consume no animal-based proteins with the exception of fish.

Following a plant-based diet will often include meat or fish in the diet, with the exceptions as listed above, regardless of varying definitions.

What about Veganism?

Vegans are considered the most drastic form of vegetarianism, refusing all animal-based proteins and by-products. This will also extend into your day-to-day life, affecting things such as the type of clothing you buy. It excludes all forms of animal exploitation and animal cruelty, including consuming honey and gelatin. While veganism is relatively new, it has gained a lot of traction over the last few years.

Both *vegetarians* and *vegans* avoid eating animal-derived products, often for similar reasons, but with the difference lying in to which extent they consider what is acceptable to consume.

Most notably, while both vegetarians and vegans exclude animal proteins for health or ethical reasons, vegans have environmental considerations. Vegetarians, on the other hand, accept the consumption of animal by-products, such as dairy and eggs, provided that the animals are kept in healthy and happy conditions.

Nutrition and Misconceptions

After some extensive research, it has been found that plant-based diets, most notably vegetarianism (as well as veganism), contain lower levels of saturated fats and cholesterol. They are also much higher in fiber.

These diets are packed with nutrient-dense foods that greatly improve the absorption of these vitamins and minerals (Craig et al., 2019). However, the risk lies in not planning the meals adequately, which could result in not having enough nutrients such as iron, calcium, and vitamin D, which are much more easily obtained if one eats larger amounts of animal sources of protein. Vegetarians and vegans both run the risk of having significantly lower levels of vitamin B_{12}; however, it is possible to maintain a healthy lifestyle following a plant-based diet, even if a person completely eliminates all animal-based food (Gibson et al., 2014).

Chapter 2: Plants and Your Health

The nutrients contained in vegetables are essential for optimal health, which is why there are many who advocate that switching to a plant-only or plant-based diet is the way to go.

Whatever your dietary considerations are, all your nutritional needs can be met on a plant-based approach, given that care is taken to balance out your meals.

Contrary to popular belief, both vegan and vegetarian diets are safe and compatible with everyone—this includes children and toddlers. Again, however, it has to be stressed that the meals have to be planned very carefully in order to ensure that the required nutrients are met for optimal health and growth. It is laborious, but the pay-off is worth the effort if you have other dietary considerations, such as allergies (Messina et al., 2001).

If not planned properly, the side effects of mineral deficiencies will not only affect physical growth but mental health as well. Vegetarian diets, as opposed to vegan diets, do consume higher quantities of calcium and vitamin B_{12} due to the fact that they would not necessarily remove dairy and eggs from their diets (the main sources of these micronutrients in aforementioned diets).

By actively focusing on nutrition, both vegans and vegetarians are able to increase the effectiveness with which their bodies are able to absorb nutrients from plant-based sources. Additionally, this strategy could be combined with the intake of supplements, especially for iron and vitamins D and B_{12} (Appleby et al., 2007). Having your blood nutrient levels measured by your general practitioner and subsequently keeping track of your daily intake, you will be able to safely and happily follow a completely plant-based diet with all the accompanying benefits.

Incorporating more plants into your diet will reduce the risk of health-related problems, such as diabetes and heart disease. It is also effective for controlling and maintaining weight.

The most important takeaway from this is that while a vegan diet is better in supporting weight loss, improving overall health, and reducing risks of many diseases, if not properly planned, there is a risk of severe nutrient deficiencies (Petre, 2016).

Chapter 3: Transitioning to a Plant-Based Diet

Switching to a new diet is not always easy. Keep in mind that transition takes time, so do not feel discouraged if you find it difficult to do so.

Below are some tips to help you transition more easily to a plant-based diet:

1. Start slow.

While it would be tempting to dive head-first into the fray, plan out a few plant-based meals and spread them throughout the week. You can continue enjoying the foods you were used to, but switch it up every so often to include this new change.

2. Reduce meat intake.

This includes processed stuff. Instead of stressing yourself out, start by simply reducing the amount of meat or meat products you consume. Small changes have far-reaching effects. Instead of a 16 oz. steak with dinner, cut it down to 8 oz. Add a large salad instead to make up the volume of your meal. Taking small steps will allow your mind and body to adjust to your new diet.

3. Commit.

Once you have had some time to try out new recipes, commit to having at least one plant-based meal per day. The easiest would be a plant-based breakfast. Go for the pancakes or smoothies contained in the recipe section of this book.

4. Protein!

Be sure to keep an eye on your protein intake. While you may be tempted to double the protein intake due to misinformation, be aware of what your body is telling you instead. Too little, and your body will tell you. Too much, and your body will do the same. Provided you are maintaining the right number of calories for your daily requirements, you should be fine. By focusing on whole, unprocessed foods, however, the risk of being deficient in this macronutrient is slim.

5. Read the labels and get to know the foods you are eating.

Even if it says "vegan" or "vegetarian" does not mean it is healthy. You may still be going "vegan" by eating ice cream and diet soda, but it is not healthy. Get familiar with how to prepare whole fruits and vegetables as this will often save you the headache of having to go over your groceries with a super fine-toothed comb.

6. Stock up on healthy snacks.

Adding healthy, plant-based snacks to your diet will help curb your cravings. Again, read the labels or make them yourself. This book has a delightful chocolate chip cookie recipe that makes it all worth it.

7. Have fun!

Keep your meals simple and fun. Go for easier recipes if you are not too familiar with the kitchen, or wrangle some friends and let them help. Scour the Internet and food blogs for new ideas if you find yourself getting bored with what you have at your disposal. The recipes in this book can be made ahead of time and frozen (Nazish, 2018).

How to Calculate Your Caloric Needs

To determine your personal caloric requirements, multiply your basal metabolic rate (BMR) with an activity factor, and either add or subtract yet another value depending on whether you want to lose, maintain, or gain weight. (More on this below.)

Your BMR refers to the energy your body requires to function over a period of 24 hours—meaning, the energy your body burns by simply being, breathing, and nothing more.

To calculate your BMR, you can either plug in your information into an online calculator or use the following equation (Ruddock, 2006):

For women:

BMR = 655 + (4.35 × weight in pounds) + (4.7 × height in inches) − (4.7 × age in years)

For men:

BMR = 66 + (6.23 × weight in pounds) + (12.7 × height in inches) − (6.8 × age in years)

Now to use it in an example, this is how you calculate BMR for an average female:

BMR = 655 + (4.35 × 147 lbs.) + (4.7 × 65 inches) − (4.7 × 27 years)

BMR = 655 + (639.45) + (305.5) − (127.9)

BMR = 1,472.05 kcal/24 hours (resting)

As you can see, the above number is what your body will need for just existing. This does not include the energy your body expends for moving, thinking, and digesting.

In order to get closer to the true number, that number will now be multiplied by an activity factor:

1. Sedentary (little or no exercise) = BMR × 1.2
2. Lightly active (light exercise, 1–3 days/week) = BMR × 1.375
3. Moderately active (moderate exercise, 3–5 days/week) = BMR × 1.55
4. Very active (hard exercise, 6–7 days a week) = BMR × 1.725
5. Extra active (very hard exercise, combined with a physically taxing job) = BMR × 1.9

In this example, the person does little exercise and has

a desk job. Therefore, the activity factor is 1.2 (little to no exercise).

So to maintain weight (or to neither lose nor gain weight), the person needs 1,472.05 × 1.2 = **1766.46 kcal/day**.

When you do your own calculations, be 100% honest with what you enter as this will affect the result.

Note: Should you wish to *gain* weight, add 500 kcal to your result—i.e., 1,766 (rounded down) + 500 = 2,266 kcal. Should you wish to *lose* weight, subtract 500 kcal from your result—i.e., 1,766 − 500 = 1,266 kcal.

Be aware! Do not reduce less than your base metabolic rate as this will negatively affect your health (as in the example above, it is just meant to illustrate the calculation). Weight loss is more effective and healthier when combined with moderate exercise.

Chapter 4: Plant-Based Foods: A Guide

Switching over from a diet you were familiar with to a new one, especially one that challenges you, can be overwhelming. The basic idea behind plant-based diets is to make vegetables central to your meals.

It does not necessarily mean you need to cut out meat-based proteins completely (it depends on how fully plant-based you are planning to go). You simply shift focus from those proteins to vegetable-based ones.

Consider this: You have been generally taught to build your meal around a protein—for example, a large steak, accompanied by roast potatoes, and a small side salad or some vegetables. In the case with a plant-based meal, you will focus your plate around your vegetables instead, with a small side dish of grilled fish or a small piece of steak.

In the event you will be going vegan, you will base your meals around your vegetables, as above, except your meat-based protein will be replaced with a plant-based one, such as tofu.

The recipes in this book are 100% vegan. Feel free to

substitute the proteins as you require for your chosen dietary requirements should you not be vegan.

What to Add to My Shopping List

Eating and maintaining a plant-based diet is not difficult. If you are new to the whole vegetable thing, it can be intimidating. Fear not! I have listed some of the food items you will need to stock up on.

Where possible, try to get fresh fruits and vegetables. If you cannot find any (i.e., out of season or inaccessible), go for frozen goods over canned. They may not last as long as the canned kind, but they will hold much more nutritional value than the canned counterparts. You will also have more variety.

You may have fresh fruit for lunchboxes, while frozen fruits for your on-the-go smoothies. Berries, bananas, and other soft fruits will last about a week in your fridge. The harder fruits will last much longer, so keep that in mind.

The recipes in this book do not necessarily require fresh

fruits, so if you need to, substitute them with the frozen ones.

Vegetables will make up the bulk of your diet when you go plant-based, whether it is vegetarian, vegan, or just as a "meat-free Monday" added to your regular routine. Vegetables such as kale, spinach, broccoli, cauliflower, and carrots are okay to buy in bulk and freeze for up to three months. Be sure to blanch them first if you buy them fresh. Other vegetables such as asparagus and eggplant are better when purchased fresh.

Many recipes call for sweet potato as a base, especially as a sort of binding agent in bread and cakes. As with the green vegetables, you can buy these in bulk, wash, peel, cut, pre-boil, and freeze them. (Just remember to keep accurate track of the dates that you freeze them at. You do not want to eat freezer-burned vegetables.)

You can use normal potatoes and other starchy vegetables such as butternut squash as well.

Rice, pasta, oats, and quinoa will help meet your fiber targets and build up the satiety levels of your meals. (If you are planning on going vegan, check the list of ingredients on the pasta as it may contain eggs or other animal by-products.)

Peas, chickpeas, lentils, peanuts, and black beans are fine either dried or canned. If you do buy the dried kind, you will need to soak them for up to twelve hours before use to rehydrate them.

Seeds and nuts are good to have around as a snack or to make your own nut butters. Many recipes will call for some of either nut butter or nut milk. Look for organic jars of the stuff if you do not want to make them yourself.

Almonds, cashews, and Macadamia nuts can be used to make either the nut butter or the nut milk. Some recipes will also call for pastes made from the soaked nuts. Tahini is also a good staple to keep around.

Your milk will include the plant-based variety—coconut, cashew, almond, etc.

Keep in mind that even if something says "vegan" or "vegetarian," it does not necessarily mean it is healthy. Read the labels if you plan on buying from the supermarket. Look for healthy fats, such as olive oil or coconut oil, for cooking. All your spices and herbs should be fresh if at all possible. If you cannot find them readily available, be sure to look at the label. Chances are some spices contain sugar as a base. Hidden sugars in foods can wreck your healthy eating habits.

For your condiments/toppings, you can find some in the sauce or canned aisle at your local supermarket. Included in this book are some recipes to make your own sauces, dips, and condiments. If you make it yourself, you know exactly what is in it—no nasty additives or non-nutritive surprises.

If you do not have the time to make them yourself or if you are in a hurry, just double-check the information label on the packaging of the product. Get familiar with the different names for sugars, genetically modified ingredients, and preservatives.

Are you looking for a cheesy kick that is not cheese? Choose nutritional yeast. It will add that cheesy flavor without compromising your diet. This is especially useful if you are going to go vegan or if you are lactose intolerant.

The biggest concern people have when switching over from eating meat on a regular basis to following a plant-based diet is where to get the protein. There are many plant-based sources you can turn to—all of which have different textures and tastes:

1. **Seitan**: This is a wheat-based protein. If you are gluten intolerant, switch it out with tempeh.

2. **Tofu**: This is bean curd made from soy milk.

3. **Tempeh**: This is fermented soybean compressed into a cake.

4. **Edamame**: This is a Japanese soybean that is still in the pod.

5. **Spelt**: This is a grain that is packed with vitamins, minerals, and nutrients. High in fiber and protein, it aids digestive health, helps lower cholesterol, and regulates glucose levels (McDonald, 2018).

6. **Green peas**: Not a lot of people love peas due to the taste and texture, but if you are allergic to soy or wheat, green peas will be the way to go.

7. **Spirulina**: This is often used more as a dietary supplement. It is recommended if you are struggling to reach your protein requirements.

8. **Amaranth and quinoa**: These are grains that are wheat-free, good for replacing other wheat-based grains such as spelt.

9. **Soy milk**: A natural by-product of making tofu. If you are allergic to soy, you can substitute with almond or rice milk.

10. **Oats and wild rice**: These are the most common fillers in a plant-based diet. They are healthy, high in protein, and easy to find in supermarkets.

Be aware of your own dietary needs. If you feel weak or achy, chances are you are either not ingesting enough calories or not enough protein. Consult your general practitioner before making any drastic changes to your diet.

You are also able to add things like coffee and tea to your diet. Preferably, these should be taken as is— meaning, no sugar, sweeteners, or milk added. However, if you cannot stand the taste of raw, natural coffee or tea, feel free to make it the way you like it.

Note, however, that switching to plant-based milk will alter the texture and taste of your hot beverage. Soy milk has a very heavy taste if added to coffee, but it tastes slightly better with more herbal type teas.

Rice milk has a rather oily base, so personally, I prefer almond milk or coconut milk in my coffee or drink it black. Rice milk is great for cooking or baking (Kubala, 2018).

Chapter 5: Recipes

The recipes that follow are 100% vegan. You can substitute certain items with animal proteins in the event that you want to switch it up. (For vegetarians, if you want to adjust your normal day-to-day eating, you can substitute your preferred source of protein).

Smoothies and Breakfast

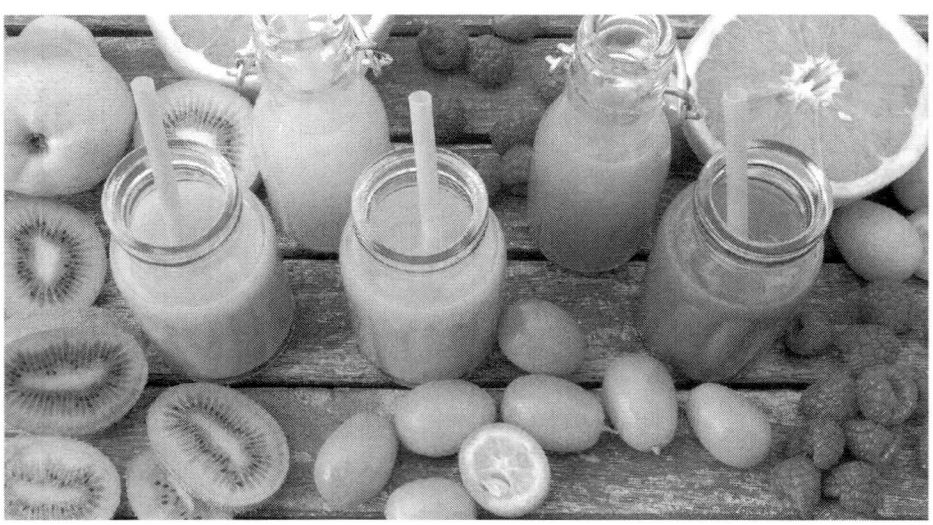

The thing to note with smoothies is that while these are healthy, they are not meant to replace regular meals.

Bananas are used as a base for the smoothies. If balanced out correctly, you will not taste the banana as much. Freezing them also has the added benefit of a nice, creamy, thick texture.

You can also freeze your bananas in ziplock bags to make preparation easier. Simply cut your ripe banana into pieces, pop into a baggie, and freeze. This will also keep the bananas from going bad on your counter. (There is only so much banana one person can eat without getting bored!)

The skin of your banana should be a bright yellow with a couple of small brown spots. The more brown spots, the sweeter the banana. However, you want the banana to be yellow, not brown, in order to maintain as much of the nutrition without the converted sugar.

These smoothies are also a little "watery," meaning thinner than you would expect. Feel free to adjust the plant-based milk in the recipe to reach the consistency you desire. Normally, it takes about half a cup less of what the recipe calls for to get a really thick, creamy texture.

If you want your smoothie to be a little sweeter than

the recipe calls for, instead of reaching for the sugar (why would you, the grainy texture ruins it!), add 2–3 drops of stevia. I find the aftertaste of sweetener lingers a little. If that does not bother you, go ahead and substitute with a liquid sweetener of your choice.

Alternatively, you can add in 3–4 pitted dates. Soft, room-temperature dates blend better than the frozen kind.

Mocha Smoothie

This recipe makes 1 smoothie.

What you need:

- 2 medium-sized bananas, sliced thickly (approx. 6–8 inches long)
- 1½ cups almond milk
- 1 tablespoon organic cocoa powder
- 2 teaspoons instant coffee powder

What to do:

1. Add the bananas and powders to a blender.

2. Pulse together a few times and add the milk a little at a time until all of it is added or the desired consistency has been reached.

3. Blend well.

Calories: 189 kcal | Carbohydrates: 35 g | Protein: 7 g | Fat: 3 g

Mint Choc-Chip Smoothie

This recipe makes 1 smoothie.

What you need:

- 2 medium-sized bananas, sliced thickly (approx. 6–8 inches long)
- 1½ cup almond milk
- 1 cup baby spinach
- 4 tablespoons fresh mint, chopped (or approx. 2 tablespoons if dried)
- 1 tablespoon chocolate chips (vegan)

- ½ teaspoon vanilla extract

What to do:

1. Add bananas and spinach to a blender.
2. Pulse together a few times until fairly mixed.
3. Add mint and chocolate chips and blend.
4. Finally, add the rest of the ingredients and blend well.

Calories: 189 kcal | Carbohydrates: 35 g | Protein: 7 g | Fat: 3 g

Blueberry Smoothie

This recipe makes 1 smoothie.

What you need:

- 2 medium-sized bananas, sliced thickly (approx. 6–8 inches long)
- 1¾ cup almond milk
- 1 cup blueberries
- ¼ cup oats

- ½ teaspoon vanilla extract

What to do:

1. Add oats to the blender and pulse a couple of times.
2. Add bananas and blueberries and whizz.
3. Add the rest of the ingredients, as well as the milk, a little at a time until all of it is added or the desired consistency has been reached.

Calories: 189 kcal | Carbohydrates: 35 g | Protein: 7 g | Fat: 3 g

Cinnamon Smoothie

This recipe makes 1 smoothie.

What you need:

- 2 medium-sized bananas, sliced thickly (approx. 6–8 inches long)
- 1½ cup almond milk
- 3–4 pitted dates

- ¼ cup oats
- ½ teaspoon vanilla extract
- ½ teaspoon ground cinnamon

What to do:

1. Add oats to the blender and pulse a couple of times.
2. Add bananas and dates and whizz.
3. Add the rest of the ingredients and the milk a little at a time until all of it is added or the desired consistency has been reached.

Calories: 189 kcal | Carbohydrates: 35 g | Protein: 7 g | Fat: 3 g

Creamy Orange Smoothie

This recipe makes 1 smoothie.

What you need:

- 2 medium-sized bananas, sliced thickly (approx. 6–8 inches long)

- 1 cup almond milk

- 1 cup of orange juice (freshly squeezed if possible)

- ½ teaspoon vanilla extract

What to do:

1. Add all the ingredients to a blender, except the milk. Using chilled orange juice (or almost frozen orange juice) will help the icy consistency, making it closer to ice cream.

2. Pulse together a few times and add the milk a little at a time until all of it is added or the desired consistency has been reached.

3. Blend well.

Calories: 189 kcal | Carbohydrates: 35 g | Protein: 7 g | Fat: 3 g

Peanut Butter Smoothie

This recipe makes 1 smoothie.

What you need:

- 2 medium-sized bananas, sliced thickly (approx. 6–8 inches long)

- 1½ cup almond milk

- 1 tablespoon organic cocoa powder

- 2 teaspoons peanut butter

- ½ teaspoon vanilla extract

What to do:

1. Add all the ingredients to a blender, except the milk.

2. Pulse together a few times and add the milk a little at a time until all of it is added or the desired consistency has been reached.

3. Blend well.

Calories: 189 kcal | Carbohydrates: 35 g | Protein: 7 g | Fat: 3 g

Berry Smoothie

This recipe makes 1 smoothie.

What you need:

- 1 medium-sized banana, sliced thickly (approx. 6–8 inches long)
- 1½ cup almond milk
- ½ cup raspberries
- ½ cup strawberries
- 2 teaspoons peanut butter

What to do:

1. Add all the ingredients to the blender, except the milk.
2. Pulse together a few times and add the milk a little at a time until all of it is added or the desired consistency has been reached.
3. Blend well.

Calories: 189 kcal | Carbohydrates: 35 g | Protein: 7 g | Fat: 3 g

Pumpkin Breakfast Cookies

Normally, cookies are a dessert or a snack, but not these chewy pumpkin breakfast cookies. They are freezable, so double the batch and freeze the dough (in a sealed ziplock bag) or bake and freeze in an airtight container. These are moist and absolutely delectable, easy to grab on the go.

This recipe makes 30 cookies.

What you need:

- 1 medium-sized banana, mashed
- ½ pumpkin, mashed
- ⅓ cup aquafaba or bean water (you can use the water that comes with canned chickpeas or use the water you boil your chickpeas in when making other recipes)
- ½ cup peanut butter
- 1½ cups oats
- 1 cup oats, ground roughly
- ¾ cup chocolate chips (you can substitute raisins

for a slightly healthier option, but let's be honest, chocolate chips are the best)

- 1 teaspoon baking powder (remember to go for gluten-free powder if there are intolerances)
- 2 teaspoons pumpkin pie spice (see recipe below)
- 1½ tablespoons maple syrup
- 2 teaspoons vanilla extract

What to do:

1. Preheat the oven to 350 degrees Fahrenheit.
2. Line a baking sheet with parchment paper.
3. Add all dry ingredients to a bowl and mix really well.
4. In a separate bowl, mix the mashed banana, pumpkin, peanut butter, syrup, and extract together, and combine thoroughly.
5. Bit by bit, add the dry ingredients to the wet and combine until everything is mixed together to form a firm dough.
6. On the prepared baking sheet, divide the dough

evenly using approximately 2 tablespoons per cookie.

7. Press the cookies slightly with a fork.

8. Bake for 15 minutes.

Calories: 30 kcal

For the pumpkin pie spice:

- 6 teaspoons cinnamon
- 1½ teaspoons ground ginger
- 1½ teaspoons nutmeg
- 1½ teaspoons allspice
- ¾ teaspoon ground cloves

Combine all the spices to a small, airtight jar. Shake until mixed well.

Pancakes

There are two secrets ingredients in this recipe: potato starch and coconut milk. You can substitute the milk with other plant-based milk, but the pancakes have a better, fluffier, creamier texture if you use canned coconut milk instead. The canned milk is thicker than those found in other packages.

The recipe also calls for pastry flour. The difference between pastry flour and regular ground flour is that pastry flour is ground much more finely. This will allow the pancakes to be extra light and fluffy—a must since this recipe has no eggs.

This recipe makes approximately 7 pancakes.

What you need:

- 1½ cups pastry flour (whole wheat)
- 3 tablespoons potato starch
- 1 tablespoon baking powder
- ½ teaspoon salt
- 1¼ cups coconut milk, room temperature, shaken well
- 2½ tablespoons maple syrup (maple syrup is preferred due to its taste, but it could be substituted by a different syrup if you prefer)
- 1 tablespoon vanilla extract

- ½ tablespoon apple cider vinegar

What to do:

1. In a large bowl, sift in your flour, starch, salt, and baking powder.

2. Combine well.

3. In a separate bowl, combine milk, vinegar, vanilla, and the syrup.

4. Add wet to dry and fold together. Using a plastic spatula, start at the bottom of the bowl and "fold" the flour over the wet ingredients. Repeat until just mixed. You do not want to overmix as this will cause the pancakes to be less fluffy.

5. Rest the batter for 15 minutes.

6. Preheat your pan at medium-low heat. You can use a non-stick spray instead of oil if you prefer. Do not use olive oil as it will alter the taste.

7. Pour ⅓ cup of batter per pancake.

8. Allow it to cook until bubbles (and little holes) start to form on top of the batter (if your pan is too warm, your pancake will burn underneath

before the bubbles form).

9. Flip your pancake over and cook for a further 1–2 minutes.

Calories: 171.5 | Fat: 2.8 g | Carbohydrates: 30.4 g | Protein: 3.8 g

Chickpea and Onion Omelet

This hearty breakfast omelet is exactly what the doctor ordered. It is vegan-friendly and super delicious. You can add in whatever other vegetables you want if onions are not your thing.

Switch it up with the seasons! Add some cubed tomatoes and basil for a summery vibe, or sliver some zucchini and spinach for a crisp, spring flavor. Go nuts!

What you need:

- 3 heaped tablespoons chickpea flour
- ½ teaspoon salt
- ½ teaspoon pepper
- 8 tablespoons water

- 1 small red onion, sliced thinly (you can use any onion you like here; the red ones are just slightly sweeter)
- ¼ cup of fresh mixed herbs (basil, spring onion (the leafy part), and thyme are some examples)
- 2 tablespoons oil

What to do:

1. Combine chickpea flour, salt, and pepper.
2. Add in the water, and whisk until you have a creamy, smooth batter.
3. For best results, fry the onions on medium heat before adding to the batter. Otherwise, if you prefer crispier onions, add them as is. Mix everything together.
4. In a large saucepan, heat a little bit of oil on medium heat. When the pan is warm, scoop all the batter into the pan.
5. Tilt the pan to allow the batter to spread. You can use a wooden spoon or rubber spatula to assist in spreading out the ingredients.

6. Cook for a few minutes with the lid removed. You do not want steam to create liquid in the pan, or else your omelet will fall apart.

7. Flip the omelet over and cook for a further 5 minutes or until hot all the way through and the omelet is firm.

8. Remove from the heat and allow to cool slightly.

9. Serve as is or with a slice of toast of your choice. You can also add it as a side to your normal breakfast if you wish for a fuller meal.

Calories: 150.5 kcal | Fat: 2.8 g | Carbohydrates: 15.4 g | Protein: 5.8 g

Gingerbread Waffles

Add some extra spice to your morning with these fragrant and spicy breakfast waffles that taste just like the holidays.

These are full of healthy ingredients with very little oil in the entire batch, and pair perfectly with fresh bananas or slices of pears. The biggest tip here is this: when the waffles are cooking in the waffle maker, steam will escape.

Do not open the waffle maker until all the steam has disappeared! It will ensure the inside is cooked through but is still light and fluffy on the inside and the outside will have a slightly crispy edge.

The batter can also double as a pancake batter if you do not have a waffle maker. You can also pour the batter into a ziplock baggie or a freezer-safe, airtight container and freeze the batter for later. Just remove from the fridge and defrost it overnight and bring to room temperature before use.

To get the perfect flour ratio, either weigh with a scale or scoop the flour into the cup with a spoon without shaking or tapping it down. Level it out with the back of a knife.

This recipe makes 6 waffles.

What you need:

- 125 g or 1 slightly heaped cup spelt flour
- 1 tablespoon ground flaxseed
- 2 teaspoons baking powder

- ¼ teaspoon baking soda
- ¼ teaspoon salt
- 1½ teaspoons cinnamon
- 2 teaspoons ground ginger
- 4 tablespoons coconut sugar or brown sugar
- 1 cup nondairy milk
- 1 tablespoon apple cider vinegar
- 2 tablespoons blackstrap molasses
- 1½ tablespoons coconut oil, melted

What to do:

1. Grease and preheat your waffle iron on setting 4 (or medium-low heat).
2. In a large bowl, sift the dry ingredients together and mix well with a wooden spoon.
3. In a separate bowl, whisk together all the wet ingredients until well combined.
4. Make a little well in the flour mixture, and slowly pour in the liquid and mix using a spoon until just

combined. Do not over mix. If you sift, you will reduce the lumps that you have, and some lumps are fine, but you want it to get to the stage that you no longer see any dry bits of flour.

5. The batter should be a thick consistency, close to a cake batter. If it is too thick, add an extra tablespoon of milk at a time and mix together.

6. Set aside for 10 minutes.

7. When your waffle iron is ready, pour in the batter and cook on medium heat until steam stops coming out of the side.

8. Carefully transfer to a plate.

9. Note: When making pancakes, pour about 3 tablespoons of batter into a preheated pan and cook over medium heat until bubbles start forming on the surface. Once you see the bubbles, flip and cook for another two minutes until the underside is darkening.

10. Serve immediately.

Calories: 200.5 kcal | Fat: 10 g | Carbohydrates: 28.4 g | Protein: 10 g

Breakfast Grits Bowl

This bowl is almost like a deconstructed breakfast sandwich, except warmer, creamier, and so very comforting.

Marinate the tofu overnight, as this will lend them that perfect flavor that binds the elements in this dish together.

This recipe makes 4 bowls.

What you need:

- 1 block extra-firm tofu, sliced into strips
- ¼ cup soy sauce, low sodium
- 1 teaspoon turmeric
- ½ teaspoon onion powder
- 1 tablespoon olive oil
- 4 servings grits (make according to the package instructions)
- ½ cup nutritional yeast
- 2 tablespoons coconut oil

- 1 medium avocado
- ¼ cup baby tomatoes, halved
- ¾ cup baby spinach
- 4 teaspoons spring onion, sliced thinly
- salt and pepper to taste

What to do:

1. Preheat the oven to 425 degrees Fahrenheit.
2. In a medium bowl, whisk together the soy sauce, turmeric, onion powder, and olive oil.
3. Add the tofu strips, and let sit for at least 15–20 minutes.
4. These are better if prepared the night before and left to marinate until morning.
5. Prepare a baking tray with non-stick spray, and arrange your tofu strips in a thin layer.
6. Bake for 15 minutes, flip, and bake for a further 15 minutes.
7. Prepare the grits as your tofu is baking.

8. You can prepare this beforehand as well, or simply time it so that the grits are ready by the time the tofu comes out of the oven.

9. When the grits are ready, stir in the nutritional yeast and coconut oil.

10. Divide between 4 bowls and top evenly with the baked tofu strips, avocado, and the other vegetables.

11. Lightly season and serve immediately.

Calories: 358 kcal

Tofu Scramble

Be careful with tofu as it is easy to over- or under-spice. This recipe is full of flavor with loads of awesome textures as it has red peppers, mushrooms, and beans. This breakfast is hearty and super filling. It is perfect for the whole family.

The extra firm silken tofu will give you the closest egg-like texture, while the firmer tofu will add a bit more chew. It's all up to you.

This recipe makes 4 servings.

What you need:

For the spice mix:

- 2 tablespoons nutritional yeast
- 1 teaspoon chili powder, ground cumin and black salt each (you can use regular salt if you cannot find black salt)
- ¾ teaspoon turmeric
- ¼ teaspoon garlic powder

For the scramble:

- 1 tablespoon olive oil
- 1½ cups button mushrooms, sliced
- 1 red pepper, chopped
- ½ onion, chopped
- 2 cloves garlic, minced
- 4–5 oz. extra firm silken tofu
- 2 cups black beans, drained and rinsed

What to do:

1. Add all of the spice mix ingredients into a bowl and stir to combine (you can double the recipe and store the rest for a later time).

2. Heat the oil over medium heat.

3. Add the onion, pepper, and garlic, and cook until fragrant and soft.

4. Add the mushrooms after 3 minutes and allow to cook in their own juices.

5. Cook for 8 minutes until everything starts to brown.

6. Break the tofu apart and add to the pan. It needs to look chunky, kind of like scrambled eggs.

7. Stir in the spice mix and black beans.

8. Cook for a further 5–8 minutes until heated through.

Calories: 175 kcal | Carbohydrates: 10 g | Protein: 14 g | Fat: 9 g

Vegan Crepes

These are thin, delicate pancakes with crispy edges—perfect as is or with whatever filling you can get your hands on.

This recipe makes 5 crepes.

What you need:

- 1 cup water
- 1 medium-sized ripe banana
- ½ cup oat flour
- ½ cup brown rice flour
- 1 teaspoon baking powder
- 1 tablespoon coconut sugar
- Pinch of salt

What to do:

1. Toss everything into a blender, and blend until smooth.

2. In a large skillet or frying pan, heat some oil on medium-high heat.

3. Pour ¼ cup of batter into the pan.

4. Tilt the pan to spread the batter around the pan as thin as possible.

5. Cook 2–3 minutes.

6. The edges will pull away from the side of the pan, and small bubbles will form when the crepe is ready to flip.

7. Slide a spatula underneath, flip, and cook for another 2 minutes.

8. Remove from the pan.

9. Repeat with the remaining batter and fill each with fruit or filling of choice. These make pretty decent desserts as well.

Calories: 100 kcal | Carbohydrates: 17 g | Protein: 5 g | Fat: 3 g

Fig Oatmeal Breakfast Bake

This recipe makes 6 servings.

What you need:

For the baked oatmeal:

- 2 cups rolled oats
- 1 cup dried figs, cut into fourths
- ½ cup cashews
- 1½ teaspoons baking powder
- ½ teaspoon cinnamon
- ¼ teaspoon salt
- 2 cups almond milk (or dairy-free milk of choice)
- ½ cup fig spread (you can cook up some figs and pulse them into a paste, adding a bit of water to thin out)
- 1 teaspoon vanilla extract

For the topping:

- ¾ cup coconut sugar
- ¾ cup flour
- ¼ cup vegan butter, softened
- 1 teaspoon cinnamon

- 1 tablespoon water

For the caramelized pears:

- 2 pears, sliced thinly
- 1 teaspoon coconut oil
- ¼ teaspoon cinnamon

What to do:

1. Preheat oven to 375 degrees Fahrenheit.
2. Grease a 9×9 cake or loaf pan.
3. In a large bowl, combine oats, dried figs, cashews, baking powder, cinnamon, and salt, mixing together well.
4. In a separate medium-sized bowl, whisk together milk, fig spread, and vanilla extract until very well combined.
5. Pour the wet ingredients, little bits at a time, into the dry ingredients, and mix well with a spoon.
6. Scoop your fig-and-oat mixture into the prepared pan and bake for 20 minutes.
7. While the mixture is baking, combine all the

topping ingredients in a medium bowl. The mixture should be well mixed but crumbly.

8. Remove the oats from the oven, and add the topping in an even layer.

9. Return to the oven and bake for an additional 10–15 minutes.

10. While your oat mixture bakes in the oven, heat the coconut oil in a large skillet on medium-high.

11. When hot, add the pears to the skillet, sprinkle with cinnamon, and cook the pears on each side for 2–3 minutes until lightly soft and colored.

12. When ready, remove the oat bake from the oven and set aside to cool for 10 minutes.

13. Top with pears and extra dried figs and serve immediately.

14. You can freeze this bake in an airtight container for easy on-the-go breakfasts.

Calories: 288 kcal | Carbohydrates: 48 g | Protein: 5 g

| Fat: 5 g

Vegan French Toast

You can use a few slices of your favorite store-bought bread or slices from the bakes you can find in this book. Either way, they are simply divine.

Day-old or stale bread works best as it will retain its form a lot better than fresh or freshly baked bread. You can even go so far as to slice up a baguette that is a few days old.

You can do one of two things: (1) You can "wet" the bread by dipping into the mixture and then transferring immediately to the pan, or (2) you can place the slice of bread in the mixture, gently submerge it in the liquid, allowing it to soak in a little of the moisture, and then transferring it to the pan. If you do this too long, the slice will tear and fall apart, but it will have a lot more moisture and taste.

Important note! This mixture is super sticky, so I recommend using a good quality non-stick frying pan and increasing the amount of butter or oil you use to coat the pan. I found keeping a little extra oil on hand and replenishing between each slice will help keep the toast from sticking and burning.

This recipe makes 4–6 servings.

What you need:

- 1 large banana
- ¾ cup full-fat coconut milk (shake the can before measuring)
- 1 tablespoon maple syrup
- 1 teaspoon vanilla extract
- 1/2 teaspoons cinnamon
- 1 tablespoon vegan butter
- 4–6 slices day-old bread (gluten-free if preferred)

What to do:

1. In a blender or food processor, add the banana, coconut milk, maple syrup, vanilla extract, and cinnamon.

2. Blend until smooth and lump-free.

3. Transfer the mixture into a shallow bowl that will fit a slice of bread of your choosing.

4. Melt the vegan butter on medium heat.

5. When the pan is hot and the butter is melted, dip a slice of bread into the batter and coat both sides (I prefer a little more flavor, so I leave the slice a few seconds per side before transferring to the pan).

6. Place the bread in the hot pan and fry for a few minutes per side or until golden brown.

7. Serve hot with maple syrup, vegan butter, and any toppings of choice.

Calories: 222 kcal | Carbohydrates: 25 g | Protein: 4 g | Fat: 12 g

Soups

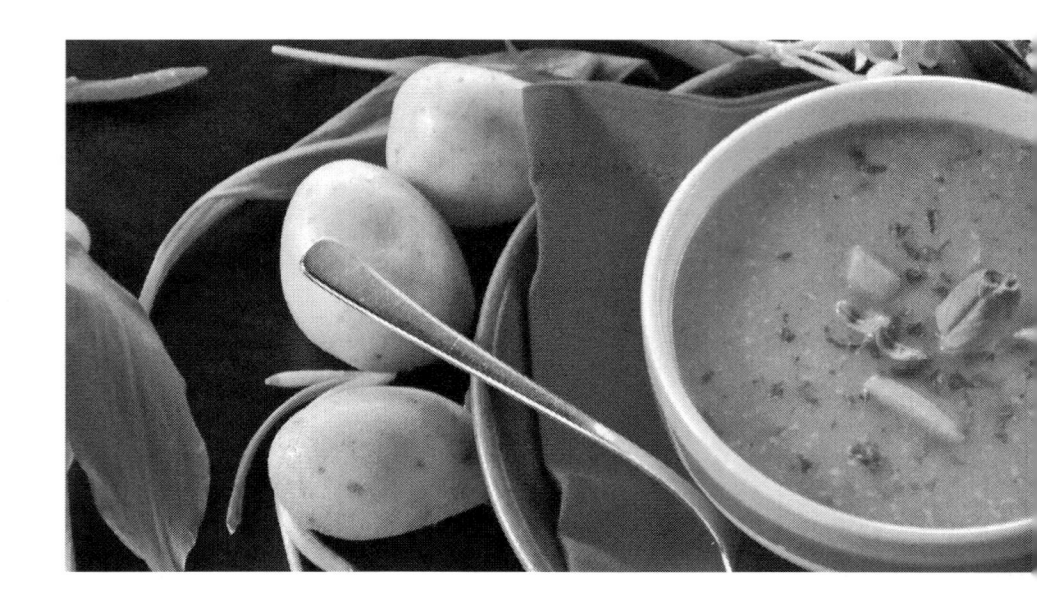

Spicy Squash Soup

If you want to be a little bit "fancy" when serving this up for your friends, you can save the cream layer floating on top of a can of coconut milk (do not shake the can before opening). You can add some ginger and lemon juice to this when beating it to add a dollop on top of your soup when serving.

This recipe makes 4 servings.

What you need:

- 2 cups silken tofu (silken tofu is softer and falls apart better than firm tofu)
- 1 can coconut milk (approx. 13 ounces)
- 1½ cups vegetable stock
- 1½ cup butternut squash, mashed
- 1 tablespoon olive oil
- 1 tablespoon lime juice
- 1 tablespoon red curry paste
- 1 teaspoon fresh ginger, grated
- ¼ cup spring onion, chopped
- 1 clove garlic, minced
- ¼ cup fresh basil, chopped (or 1 tablespoon dried)
- 1 teaspoon ground cumin
- 1 teaspoon coriander
- 1 teaspoon brown sugar (brown is better than white)
- ¼ teaspoon chili flakes

- ½ salt

What to do:

1. In a large, deep-bottomed pot, heat the oil over medium heat.
2. Add the curry paste, ginger, garlic, and spices. Cook until fragrant.
3. Whisk coconut milk until emulsified and add to the pan.
4. Add in the stock and butternut and bring to a boil.
5. Reduce and simmer 10 minutes.
6. Allow to cool slightly, and with an immersion blender, blend until smooth.
7. In a separate pan, add tofu, lime juice, and salt. Stir on medium heat until heated through.
8. Add in the basil and spring onion.
9. Cook for a minute and divide between 4 bowls.
10. Top evenly with the soup base and serve.

Calories: 250 kcal | Fat: 11 g | Protein: 9 g | Carbohydrate: 33 g

Tomato Soup

This recipe makes 4 servings.

What you need:

- 2 cups roasted tomato (canned is easier but sometimes a little more acidic to taste, or you can pan or fire-roast them yourself)
- 1 cup vegetable stock
- ⅓ cup coconut cream
- ¾ cup onion, finely chopped
- ⅓ cup carrot, finely chopped
- 6 garlic cloves, crushed
- 2 tablespoons tomato paste
- ¼ teaspoon salt
- ½ teaspoon paprika
- ¼ teaspoon ground cumin
- ¼ teaspoon cayenne pepper
- ½ cup vegan cheese, grated (Violife or similar

that grates pretty easily)

- ½ fine breadcrumbs

What to do:

1. In a large saucepan, heat the olive oil over medium heat.
2. Add onions, carrots, and garlic. Fry until fragrant and the onion is soft and lightly golden.
3. Stir in the tomato paste.
4. Add tomatoes and stock and bring to a simmer and allow to cook for approximately 5 minutes before adding the cream and salt.
5. Allow it to cool slightly. Add the mixture to a blender and blend until smooth.
6. Divide into 4 bowls.
7. In a separate pan, combine breadcrumbs, cheese, and spices, heating until the cheese starts to melt.
8. Separate the mixture into 12 even heaps, flattening with the back of the spoon.

9. Cook until brown and crispy.

10. Serve the cooled crisps with the soup.

Calories: 326 | Fat: 20 g | Protein: 9 g | Carbohydrates: 28 g

Mushroom Soup

For the best results, soak your mushrooms overnight.

This recipe makes 4 servings.

What you need:

- 4 cups mushrooms, dried (porcini or shiitake mushrooms)
- 3 tablespoons olive oil
- 1 cup fresh button mushrooms
- 1 cup potato, chopped
- 1½ cups onion, finely chopped
- 1 cup celery, finely chopped
- 2 cloves garlic, minced

- 3 tablespoons apple cider vinegar
- ½ teaspoon dried thyme
- ½ teaspoon dill
- ½ teaspoon ground white pepper
- 2 tablespoons flour or potato starch
- 1 bay leaf
- Pinch of cayenne pepper and salt
- 6–8 cups of water

What to do:

1. Soak the dried mushrooms in 2 cups warm water. Keep the water as stock for the soup.

2. Coarsely chop the mushrooms after gently squeezing the water from them and set aside. Strain the mushroom liquid and add the water and set aside.

3. In a deep pan, heat the oil and add the onions, celery, and garlic.

4. Cook until the onions are slightly soft and add the mushrooms. Cook approximately 10 minutes.

5. Add herbs and spices and continue stirring.

6. Sprinkle the potato starch over the mixture until the liquid thickens.

7. Add the mushrooms and the liquid to the pot, stirring constantly and scraping the sides. Add the bay leaf and cook for 15 minutes.

8. Add the potatoes and reduce the heat. Cook 45 minutes and remove the bay leaf. Allow to cool before adding the vinegar.

9. Blend the mixture until smooth with an immersion blender.

Calories: 100 kcal | Fat: 4 g | Protein: 4 g | Carbohydrates: 13 g

Noodle Soup

What you need:

- 1½ cups carrots, sliced
- 1½ cups celery stalks, sliced
- 2½ cups potatoes, diced

- 1 cup onion, diced
- 3 cloves garlic, minced
- 6 cups vegetable stock (low sodium preferred)
- 1 teaspoon thyme
- 1 teaspoon sea salt
- 1 tablespoon Italian herbs
- 2 tablespoons nutritional yeast
- 2 cups brown rice noodles

(Be sure to taste the soup after cooking. You may need to add more seasonings to your taste.)

What to do:

1. Add the stock to a large pot and bring it to the boil.
2. Add the herbs and spices and stir to dissolve.
3. Add all the vegetables and the nutritional yeast and bring to a boil.
4. Reduce the heat and simmer for 15 minutes.
5. Add the potatoes and cook until soft.

6. Finally, add the pasta and cook for 10 minutes.

7. Serve.

Calories: 162.3 kcal | Fat: 1.9 g | Protein: 3.4 g | Carbohydrates: 33.5 g

Salads and Sides

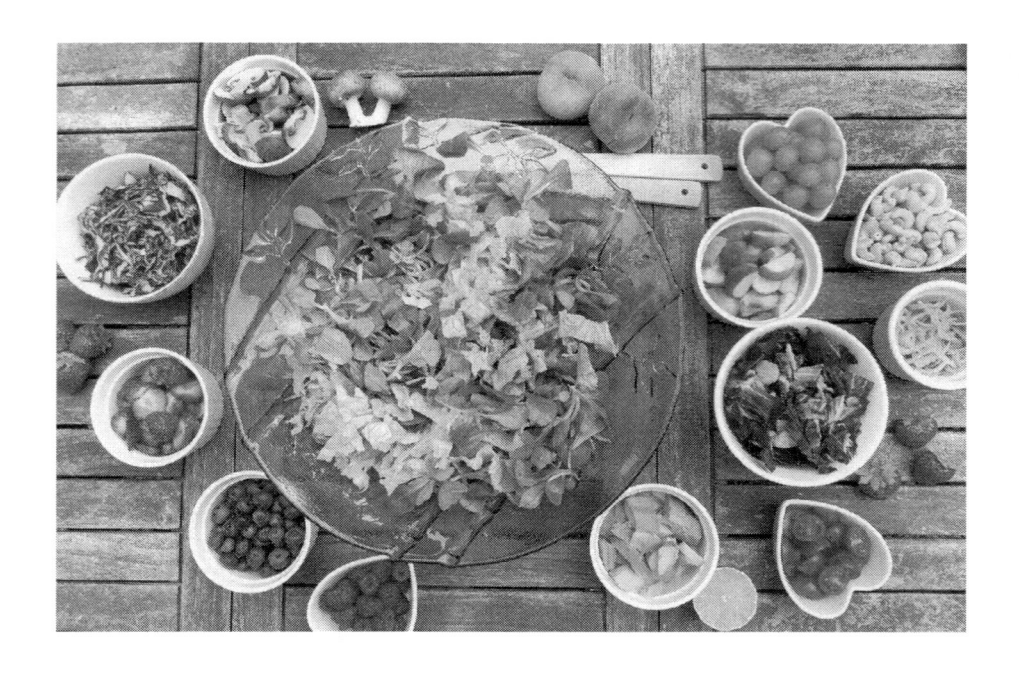

Cinnamon-Apple Bread

This sweet bread is delicious with home-made nut butters or just as a side to a spicy soup. Substituting a different flour will change the texture of the bread. This is useful if you want to turn this recipe into delightful breakfast muffins. This recipe is a little finicky, so be sure to follow the list of ingredients to ensure success.

This recipe makes 1 loaf.

What you need:

- 1¾ cups white rice flour (only use this flour if you are making it as a bread; using brown flour makes it crumblier and dry)
- ¼ cup potato starch
- ¾ cup light brown sugar
- 1 tablespoon baking powder
- 2 teaspoons ground cinnamon
- ½ teaspoon sea salt
- 1½ cup applesauce
- ¼ cup aquafaba
- ¼ cup almond butter

To make the cinnamon sugar layer:

- 4 tablespoons brown sugar
- 1½ ground cinnamon

What to do:

1. Preheat an oven to 350 degrees Fahrenheit.
2. Grease a loaf pan with oil and set aside.

3. In a large bowl, add the dry ingredients together and mix well.

4. Add in the applesauce, aquafaba, and almond butter, mixing until smooth.

5. Pour half the mixture into the prepared pan, making sure to spread the layer out evenly.

6. Sprinkle half the cinnamon-sugar mixture over the batter.

7. Pour the rest of the batter into the pan and sprinkle the cinnamon-sugar mixture.

8. Bake for an hour, keeping an eye on the bread to make sure it does not burn. You can test it by inserting a toothpick. Remove the pan from the oven as soon as the toothpick comes out dry.

9. Allow to cool completely before slicing.

Calories: 308 kcal | Carbohydrates: 40 g | Protein: 3 g | Fat: 16 g

Zucchini Bread

This bread tastes as close to banana bread as you can

get without bananas. Sweet with a hint of cinnamon, this bread is lovely when heated slightly with a dollop of almond butter.

This recipe makes 1 loaf.

What you need:

- 2 cups flour (all-purpose preferred, or you can substitute with finely ground almond flour)
- 1 cup white sugar (it is sweeter, but you can use a light-brown sugar)
- 2 teaspoons baking powder
- 1 teaspoon ground cinnamon
- ½ teaspoon salt
- ¾ cup almond milk
- ¾ cup coconut oil
- 1 tablespoon lemon juice
- 1 teaspoon vanilla extract
- 1½ cups zucchini, grated
- ½ cup walnuts, roughly chopped

What to do:

1. Preheat the oven to 350 degrees Fahrenheit.
2. Line a loaf pan with parchment paper and set aside.
3. Carefully combine all the dry ingredients together in a large bowl (leaving the walnuts aside).
4. In a separate bowl, mix together all the wet ingredients, except the grated zucchini.
5. Combine the wet and dry ingredients until just mixed.
6. Add in the zucchini and walnuts until well combined. Be careful not to overmix.
7. Pour batter into the loaf pan and bake for 80 minutes until golden.
8. Allow to cool before removing from the pan or slicing.

Calories: 298 kcal | Carbohydrates: 34 g | Protein: 3 g | Fat: 16 g

Tortilla Roll-Ups

This recipe makes 16 servings.

What you need:

- 1 recipe sour cream (see below for vegan recipe)
- ½ red bell pepper, cut into strips
- ½ yellow bell pepper, cut into strips
- 2 medium-sized carrots, cut into thin strips
- 3 small radishes, cut into really thin strips
- 1 cucumber, cut into thin strips
- 2 cups arugula, washed, shredded
- 8 large tortilla sheets

What to do:

1. On each tortilla, spread 3 tablespoons of sour cream.
2. Carefully divide the sliced vegetables between the 8 tortillas.
3. Layer the vegetables over the sour cream and

sprinkle with arugula.

4. Wrap the tortillas as tightly as possible and cut in half.

Calories: 165 kcal | Fat: 7 g | Carbohydrates: 22 g | Protein: 5 g

Coconut Potatoes

This recipe makes 5 servings.

What you need:

- 5 cups baby potatoes
- 1¾ cups coconut milk
- ¼ cup flour
- 4 cloves garlic, crushed
- 1 tablespoon fresh thyme
- ¾ teaspoon salt
- ¼ teaspoon black pepper
- ¼ teaspoon nutmeg

What to do:

1. Preheat your oven to 400 degrees Fahrenheit.
2. Whisk together all your ingredients except the potatoes and pour into a deep oven-safe dish.
3. Add in the potatoes, mixing it into the cream mixture.
4. Cover with foil and bake for 50 minutes until the potatoes are soft.

Calories: 187 kcal | Fat: 7 g | Carbohydrates: 22 g | Protein: 6 g

Grilled Butternut Squash

This recipe makes 2 servings.

What you need:

- 1 large butternut squash
- 1 tablespoon olive oil
- black pepper and nutmeg to taste

What to do:

1. Peel the squash, cut it into ½ inch slices, and clean out the seeds.

2. Brush olive oil on both sides of the slices.

3. Heat a griddle pan on medium-high heat.

4. Grill the slices for 5 minutes.

5. Sprinkle each slice with pepper and nutmeg.

6. Serve as is or with a homemade sauce.

Calories: 143 kcal | Fat: 5 g | Carbohydrates: 20 g | Protein: 3 g

Chili

Traditionally a main dish, this is used to complement the lighter meals as a side.

This recipe makes 8 servings.

What you need:

- 1½ tablespoons olive oil
- 2 cups onion, diced
- 2 tablespoons garlic, minced

- 2 medium-sized jalapeños, deseeded, chopped
- 1 cup celery, finely chopped
- 1 large bell pepper, diced (roasted pepper adds an extra level of flavor)
- 3 cups diced tomatoes
- 1 cup vegetable stock
- 6 tablespoons tomato puree
- 1½ cup cooked kidney beans
- 1½ cup navy beans
- 2 tablespoons chili powder
- 2 teaspoons ground cumin
- 1 teaspoon oregano
- Salt to taste
- Optional hot sauce for heat

What to do:

1. Heat the oil over medium heat and fry the onion and garlic until soft.

2. Add the jalapeños, celery, and bell pepper and cook until soft.

3. Lightly season with salt, and add the tomatoes, stock, and tomato paste.

4. Turn up the heat to bring the pot to a boil.

5. Add the beans and spices, and cook uncovered for 15 minutes.

6. Serve with sour cream and chopped spring onion and cilantro.

Calories: 180 kcal | Fat: 4 g | Carbohydrates: 28 g | Protein: 8 g

Avo and Noodle Salad

This salad is perfect both as a light meal and a main meal. Be sure to keep an eye on the soba noodles as they tend to cook really fast. Rinse in cold water to stop the cooking process. The noodles should not be overcooked as it could ruin the overall texture of the salad.

This recipe makes 4 servings.

What you need:

For the dressing:

- 2 tablespoons sesame oil
- 2 tablespoons soy sauce
- 1 tablespoon rice vinegar
- 1 teaspoon brown sugar
- 1 teaspoon hot mustard
- 1 teaspoon fresh ginger, grated
- 1 clove garlic, crushed
- Pinch of salt

For the salad:

- 2 large carrots, peeled and ribboned
- 2 cups fresh snow peas
- 2 cups fresh asparagus
- 2 cups uncooked soba noodles
- ¼ cup fresh basil, shredded

What to do:

For the dressing:

1. Whisk all the ingredients together and set aside.

For the salad:

1. Bring a large pot of water to a boil and add the peas and asparagus.
2. Cook vegetables for 2 minutes and remove from the heat, draining and rinsing with cold water.
3. After the vegetables are cool, add them and the carrots to the dressing and set aside.
4. Add the noodles to the boiling water and cook for approximately 5 to 6 minutes.
5. Rinse with cold water.
6. Add noodles to the other ingredients and toss well.
7. Serve.

Calories: 321 kcal | Fat: 8 g | Protein: 10 g | Carbohydrates: 55 g

Fig and Arugula Salad

This salad is simple and sweet, easy as a light side dish.

This recipe makes 4 servings.

What you need:

For the dressing:

- ⅛ teaspoons cayenne pepper
- 2 tablespoons olive oil
- ½ teaspoon salt
- 2 teaspoons balsamic vinegar
- ½ teaspoon maple syrup

For the salad:

- ½ cup walnuts, halved
- 2 cups cooked chickpeas
- 1½ cup fresh arugula, shredded
- ½ cup figs, quartered
- 1 cup of carrots, shaved

- ¾ cups crumbly vegan cheese

What to do:

For the dressing:

1. Whisk all the ingredients together in a bowl and set aside.

For the salad:

1. Preheat oven to 375 degrees Fahrenheit.
2. Mix together walnuts, cayenne pepper, and some olive oil and bake until golden.
3. Remove from oven and set aside.
4. Toss together chickpeas, arugula, figs, and carrots in a bowl. Drizzle with the dressing.
5. Add walnuts and cheese and serve.

Calories: 403 kcal | Fat: 24 g | Protein: 13 g | Carbohydrates: 35 g

Spring Salad

Use a soft vegan cheese to make the herbed cheese roll

and use plastic wrap to bind the herbs together and make rolling and subsequent slicing easier.

This recipe makes 4 servings.

What you need:

- 1½ cups fresh asparagus, cut into thirds
- 1 cup green peas
- 3 cups fresh baby spinach
- 1 cup radishes, thinly sliced
- ¼ cup roasted almonds
- 1 tablespoon parsley and chives each, chopped
- 2 cups soft vegan cheese (you can use a goat cheese log if you prefer)
- 1 teaspoon lime zest
- 1 teaspoon wholegrain mustard
- 2 tablespoons lime juice
- 1 teaspoon molasses or a similar syrup
- 1 teaspoon fresh mint

- ¼ teaspoon black pepper
- ¼ teaspoon salt
- 2½ teaspoons olive oil

What to do:

1. Bring water to boil, and then add the asparagus and peas. Cook until just tender.
2. Remove from pot and rinse with cold water to halt the cooking process. Drain and set aside to dry.
3. Place a sheet of plastic wrap on your work surface, and sprinkle parsley and chives mixture in the center.
4. Carefully lay your vegan cheese over the herbs, making sure to coat the whole thing.
5. Using the plastic wrap, gently roll the cheese into a thick log (approximately 4 inches long) and refrigerate.
6. To make the dressing, whisk together the zest, molasses, lime juice, mint, salt and pepper, and mustard.
7. Once combined, carefully whisk in the oil until all

of it has been mixed together.

8. Pour dressing over the spinach, adding in the asparagus, radishes, and peas. Toss well.

9. Cut ½-inch slices of your herbed cheese roll and add to the salad.

10. Top with roasted almonds and sprinkle with mint leaves.

Calories: 245 kcal | Fat: 18 g | Protein: 10 g | Carbohydrates: 14 g

Summer Salad

This salad is a little more filling, but it is just as delicious as an accompaniment to a hearty lasagna.

This recipe makes 4 servings.

What you need:

- 1½ cups of tempeh, cut into cubes
- 1 cup fresh asparagus, cleaned and trimmed
- 3 cups baby arugula

- 2 cups baby kale
- 2 cups spinach
- 1 cup radishes, grated
- 1 cup baby tomatoes, halved
- 2 cloves of garlic, minced
- ½ teaspoon salt
- ½ teaspoon black pepper
- 2 tablespoons olive oil
- 3 teaspoons lemon juice
- 1½ teaspoons tahini
- 1 teaspoon brown sugar
- 2 tablespoons beet kvass (this is a sort of fermented beverage; you can substitute it with unsweetened kombucha)

What to do:

1. Preheat oven to 375 degrees Fahrenheit.
2. In a small bowl, combine the tempeh, garlic, pepper and salt, oil, and lemon juice.

3. Mix until thoroughly covered and pour onto a prepared baking sheet.

4. Bake for 20 minutes, shaking the tray at 10 minutes.

5. While the tempeh is in the oven, bring a large pot of water to a boil and cook the asparagus until just tender.

6. Rinse with ice-cold water to halt the cooking process. Drain.

7. For the dressing, combine 1 tablespoon of oil, 2 teaspoons of lemon juice, and salt in a large bowl.

8. Whisk in the kvass, tahini, and sugar. If you want a thinner dressing, whisk in about 2 tablespoons of water until the desired consistency has been reached.

9. Add all the vegetables together in the dressing bowl and toss well.

Calories: 259 kcal | Fat: 17 g | Protein: 16 g | Carbohydrates: 15 g

Chickpea Meatballs and Romaine Salad

Serve as a lovely salad or as a side. The "meatballs" are delicious cold or hot.

This recipe makes 4 servings.

What you need:

- 3 cups romaine lettuce, shredded
- 1 cup cucumber, chopped
- 1 cup baby tomatoes, halved
- 1 cup red onion, thinly sliced
- 1 cup parsley, whole
- 2 cups cooked chickpeas (fresh is better, but canned is fine)
- ½ cup breadcrumbs
- 3 cloves garlic, crushed
- 3 tablespoons tahini
- 3 tablespoons lemon juice
- 1½ tablespoons water

- ¼ teaspoon salt
- ¼ teaspoon black pepper
- ¼ cup olive oil
- 1 tablespoon nut butter of choice (this is used as a binding agent; you can use 1 large egg if you wish instead, or cooked sweet potato, mashed)
- 1 teaspoon ground cumin
- 1 teaspoon paprika

What to do:

1. In a large bowl, combine lettuce, parsley, cucumber, tomatoes, and onions and set aside.
2. In a separate bowl, whisk together 1 teaspoon of crushed garlic, lemon juice, water, salt, and pepper.
3. Add in the oil and tahini and whisk thoroughly. Set aside.
4. In a food processor, add chickpeas and remaining garlic, and pulse until smooth.

5. Add in the rest of the spices, breadcrumbs, and 2 tablespoons tahini.

6. Scoop the mixture into a bowl and add the binding agent.

7. Form into balls of approximately 1 tablespoon each, and brown the balls in a pan over medium-high heat until crisp.

8. Serve with the salad, and drizzle generously with the tahini dressing.

Calories: 424 kcal | Fat: 26 g | Protein: 14 g | Carbohydrate: 36 g

Roasted Summer Veggies

This recipe makes 4 servings.

What you need:

- ¾ cup uncooked farro (emmer or spelt)
- 2 cups fresh green beans, trimmed and halved
- 1½ cups fresh asparagus, halves
- 1½ cup baby arugula

- ½ cup carrots, diced
- ¼ cup spring onion, quartered
- 3 tablespoons olive oil
- 3 teaspoons salt
- 3 teaspoons pepper
- 2 tablespoons white wine vinegar (or apple cider vinegar)
- 2 teaspoons fresh tarragon
- ½ teaspoon lemon zest
- ¼ cup almonds, roasted
- ¼ cup vegan cheese, shredded

What to do:

1. Preheat oven to 400 degrees Fahrenheit.
2. On high heat, bring water to a boil, stirring in the farro following the cooking instructions.
3. Just before the farro is done, add the green beans, and cook until just tender.
4. Drain farro mixture and rinse with cold water.

5. In a separate mixing bowl, combine together the asparagus, carrots, and spring onions with salt and oil and bake for 20 minutes.

6. To make the sauce, whisk vinegar tarragon, zest, salt, pepper, and ¼ cup olive oil until mixed.

7. Pour over the cooked farro and combine well with the arugula and other vegetables.

8. Divide between serving bowls, and top evenly with roasted almonds and shredded cheese.

Calories: 365 kcal | Fat: 28 g | Protein: 9 g | Carbohydrate: 27 g

Roasted Cauli-Wedges

This recipe makes 8 wedges.

What you need:

- 1 large head cauliflower
- ½ teaspoon ground turmeric
- ½ teaspoon chili flakes
- 1 tablespoon lemon juice

- 2 tablespoons olive oil

What to do:

1. Preheat oven to 350 degrees Fahrenheit.

2. Prepare a baking tray with parchment paper.

3. Clean the cauliflower head by removing the leaves and trimming the stem.

4. Slice the head into 8 equal pieces.

5. Brush generously with olive oil and sprinkle spices on both sides.

6. Pack onto the tray and bake until tender and slightly browned.

7. To serve, drizzle with lemon juice.

Calories: 98 kcal | Fat: 18 g | Protein: 3 g | Carbohydrate: 5 g

Roasted Pumpkin and Brussels Sprouts

This recipe makes 4–6 servings.

What you need:

- 1 medium-sized pumpkin (the kind used for making pies, approx. 3 pounds), peeled and cut into cubes (if you want, you can buy pre-cleaned and packaged pumpkin)
- 1 pound fresh Brussels sprouts, halved
- 4 cloves garlic, thinly sliced
- ⅓ cup olive oil
- 2 tablespoons balsamic vinegar
- 1 teaspoon salt
- 1 teaspoon pepper
- 2 tablespoons fresh parsley

What to do:

1. Preheat oven to 400 degrees Fahrenheit.
2. In a large bowl, combine vegetables and garlic. Whisk together oil, vinegar, salt, and pepper, and pour over the vegetables.
3. Toss to coat, transferring to a prepared baking tray.
4. Bake for 40 minutes or until vegetables are

tender.

5. Allow to cool and sprinkle with parsley. Serve.

Calories: 152 kcal | Fat: 9 g | Carbohydrates 17 g | Protein: 4 g

Sun-Dried Tomato Quiche

Creamy, rich, and decadent, this filling is baked into a flaky pie crust, and it is perfect for any meal and any occasion.

This recipe makes 8 servings.

What you need:

For the crust:

- 1½ cups all-purpose flour
- ½ teaspoon salt
- ½ cup non-dairy butter
- 2–3 tablespoons cold water

For the filling:

- 1 tablespoon coconut or vegetable oil

- ¼ cup onion, minced
- 1 cup asparagus, chopped
- 3 tablespoons dried tomatoes, chopped
- 14 ounces firm tofu, drained
- 3 tablespoons nutritional yeast
- 1 tablespoon nut milk of choice
- 1 tablespoon all-purpose flour
- 1 teaspoon dried onion
- 1 teaspoon spicy mustard
- 2 teaspoons lemon juice
- ½ teaspoon sea salt
- ½ teaspoon turmeric
- ½ teaspoon liquid smoke
- 3 tablespoons basil, chopped
- ⅓ cup vegan mozzarella cheese, shredded
- salt and pepper to taste

What to do:

1. Preheat the oven to 350 degrees Fahrenheit.

2. Prepare one 9-inch pie pan or 8.5-inch mini quiche dishes and set aside.

3. For the crust, combine flour and salt in a bowl, mixing well. Add butter in small clumps and rub in with your fingers until it resembles small pea-sized pieces and everything is thoroughly mixed in. Add cold water and transfer to a floured surface. Mix together well. It will be rather dry but should stick together when squeezed together in your hands.

4. Press into the prepared pan and bake for 10 minutes. Remove from oven and set aside to cool.

5. To make the quiche filling, heat 1 tablespoon of oil over medium heat. Add onions and cook until translucent. Add asparagus and tomatoes, cooking until asparagus becomes tender. Remove from heat and set aside.

6. In a food processor, add in the tofu, yeast, milk, flour, onions, liquid smoke, lemon juice, and spices. Blend until the mixture is completely smooth.

7. Add mixture to the asparagus mixture and combine together with fresh basil and vegan cheese, stirring until combined. Season with salt and pepper to taste.

8. Spoon filling into pie dish (be sure that the crust has cooled completely), smoothing over the top. Bake for 30–45 minutes.

9. If using small quiche bowl, divide mixture evenly and bake for 15–20 minutes or until top has browned slightly. (You can also test by piercing the middle with a knife or knitting needle. It should come away clean and dry.)

10. Remove from heat and allow to cool for at least 20 minutes before serving.

Calories: 221 kcal | Fat: 12 g | Carbohydrates: 22 g | Protein: 4 g

Main Dishes

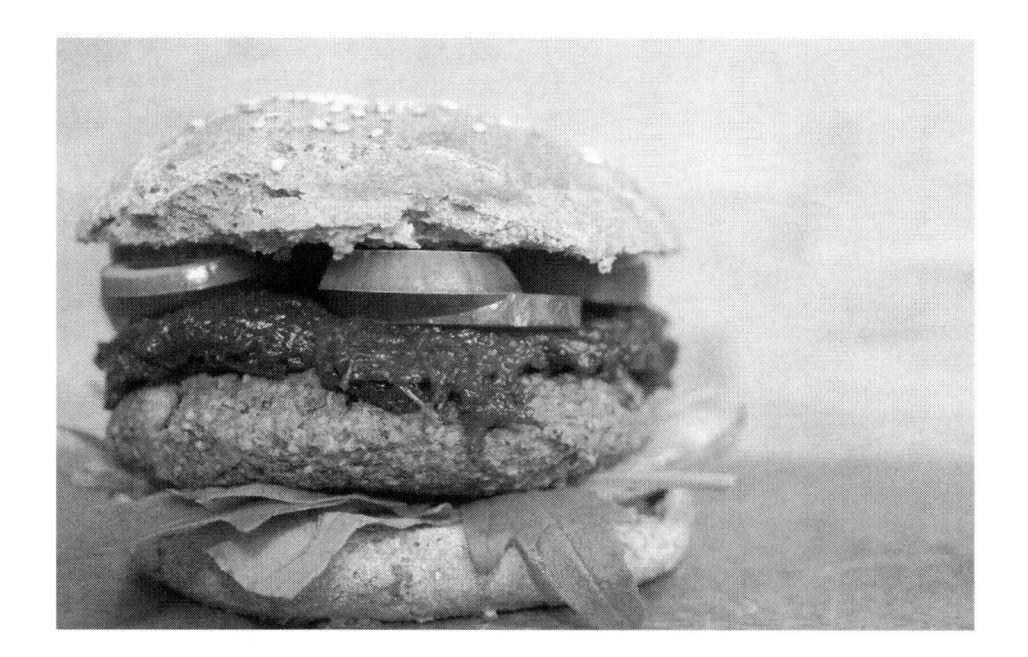

Sloppy Joe

Serve on a toasted bun as is or with your favorite toppings. This recipe is saucy and delicious. Do note that if you cannot find vegetable mince (vegan mince), you can use dried or frozen soya mince. The dried mince will require approximately 1–2 cups of extra stock.

This recipe makes about 6 Joes.

What you need:

- 1 tablespoon olive oil
- 1 medium onion, chopped
- 2 cloves garlic, crushed
- ¾ cup vegan mince
- 1½ cups chopped tomatoes (or 1 can if you prefer)
- 1 cup red bell pepper, chopped
- 1 teaspoon paprika
- 1 teaspoon ground cumin
- 1 teaspoon onion powder
- ¼ cup vegetable stock
- 3 tablespoons tomato puree
- 1 tablespoon vinegar

- 1 tablespoon maple syrup

- Salt and pepper to taste

What to do:

1. In a large frying pan, heat the oil and cook the onion and garlic until fragrant.

2. Add the bell pepper and cook for a further 3 minutes before adding in the herbs and spices.

3. Adding in the stock, puree, vinegar, and syrup, cook the mince on medium heat 15–20 minutes until the sauce thickens.

Calories: 175 kcal | Fat: 7.6 g | Carbohydrates: 21.5 | Protein: 10

Zucchini Lasagna

For this filling dinner, traditional lasagna sheets have been replaced by thinly sliced zucchini. A large zucchini yields larger "sheets" and lends a more authentic feel. You can also substitute the zucchini with eggplant or sweet potato or vegan (and gluten-free) lasagna sheets at the supermarket (if you can find them).

If you substitute the Macadamia nuts with tofu, ensure that it is the extra-firm kind and not silken. Adjust your seasonings as well, almost doubling the yeast and basil.

This recipe makes 9 servings.

What you need:

- 3 cups raw Macadamia nuts (you can use 2 cups of extra-firm tofu as well, but make sure it has been drained well)
- 2 teaspoons nutritional yeast
- 2 teaspoons dried oregano
- ½ cup fresh basil, chopped
- 2 tablespoons lemon juice
- ½ cup water
- 1 tablespoon olive oil
- salt and pepper to taste
- ¼ cup vegan cheese, plus ½ cup for topping
- 4 cups marinara sauce (you can buy a jar of your favorite at your local market)

- 3 large zucchini, thinly sliced

What to do:

1. Preheat oven to 375 degrees Fahrenheit.

2. In a food processor, blend down the macadamia nuts until a very fine meal is achieved, using a spatula to scrape down the sides.

3. Add in the rest of the ingredients, except the zucchini, sauce, and ½ cup of cheese. Season to taste (the aim is to get a well-blended, thick paste).

4. In an oven-safe dish, layer a cup of sauce, and lay down an even layer of zucchini.

5. Use a tablespoon to scoop the ricotta mixture and spread evenly.

6. Layer with sauce, zucchini, and cheese mixture until all your mixture is used.

7. Add a generous layer of cheese on top and cover with foil and bake for 45 minutes.

8. Remove the foil and bake a further 15 minutes.

9. Allow to cool slightly and serve immediately with

additional vegan Parmesan cheese and fresh basil.

Calories: 338 kcal | Fat: 34 g | Carbohydrates: 10 g | Protein: 4.7 g

Crispy Tofu Stir-Fry

Crisp your tofu beforehand in the oven. This will ensure that it retains its crispiness when you add it to the sauce, adding a lovely extra level to the dish.

This recipe makes 6 servings.

What you need:

- 1½ cups extra-firm tofu, drained
- 1 tablespoon sesame oil
- 1 head cauliflower, shredded
- 1 cup baby bok choy
- ¼ cup onion, slivered
- ¼ cup bell peppers and carrots, thinly sliced
- 2 cloves garlic, minced

For the sauce:

- 1½ tablespoons sesame oil
- ¼ cup soy sauce
- ¼ cup brown sugar
- ½ teaspoon chili sauce
- 2½ tablespoons nut butter of choice

What to do:

1. Preheat the oven to 400 degrees Fahrenheit.
2. After the tofu has been drained properly, cut your tofu into cubes.
3. Blend oil and garlic together and coat the tofu thoroughly.
4. Bake for 25 minutes until crispy.
5. Whisk together the ingredients for the sauce and set aside. You can add salt and pepper to taste. Adjust the amount of chili sauce for either more or less heat.
6. When the tofu is completely cooled, add to the bowl containing the sauce and allow to marinate

for 15 minutes.

7. For the rest of the vegetables, heat oil in a large frying pan on medium heat and add the vegetables and shredded cauliflower.

8. Cook until the vegetables are just soft, and spoon in the tofu, leaving the sauce in the bowl.

9. Remove from heat and serve with leftover sauce.

Calories: 280 kcal | Fat: 34 g | Carbohydrates: 10 g | Protein: 4.7 g

Mac and Cheese

This vegan-friendly mac and cheese is an easy dupe for the real deal. Incredibly cheesy and delicious, this recipe makes a filling meal. Soaking the cashews makes them easier to blend up; however, if you have a powerful-enough food processor, you can omit soaking altogether.

This recipe makes 2–4 servings.

What you need:

- 1 cup dried macaroni (your favorite kind)

- 1½ cups broccoli florets
- 1½ tablespoons olive oil
- 1 cup onion, chopped
- 1 cup potato, grated
- 3 cloves garlic, crushed
- ½ teaspoon garlic
- ½ teaspoon onion
- ½ teaspoon mustard powder
- Salt and pepper to taste
- ⅔ cup cashews, soaked
- 2 teaspoons apple cider vinegar
- Chili flakes to taste

What to do:

1. Follow the on-pack instructions to cook the macaroni, adding in the broccoli 2 minutes before the pasta is fully cooked.
2. Rinse in cool water and set aside.

3. In a separate pan, heat the oil. Add the onion and cook until translucent.

4. Add in the potato, garlic, and spices, constantly stirring to prevent burning.

5. Add the cashews and a cup of water, cooking until the potatoes are cooked thoroughly.

6. Allow to cool slightly and transfer into a blender, adding in the yeast, salt, and pepper.

7. Blend until smooth, adding in extra water little bits at a time to get the consistency you require.

8. Divide the pasta and pour the sauce over the top.

9. You can sprinkle extra-vegan cheese if you want an extra stringy cheesy base.

Calories: 506 kcal | Fat 21.7 g | Carbohydrate 66.5 g | Protein 18.3 g

Avo-Kale-Veggie Bowl

This recipe makes 4 servings.

What you need:

- 3 cups sweet potatoes, peeled, diced
- 3 tablespoons olive oil
- 1 teaspoon salt
- 1 teaspoon pepper
- 1 teaspoon chili powder
- 1 bell pepper, quartered and cleaned
- ½ cup almonds, chopped
- 2 teaspoons lime zest
- ½ teaspoon brown sugar
- 2 tablespoons lime juice
- 2 cups quinoa, cooked
- 4 cups baby kale
- 2 cups avocado, sliced
- ¼ cup shredded vegan cheese

What to do:

1. Preheat oven to 400 degrees Fahrenheit.
2. Prepare a baking sheet with parchment paper.

3. In a bowl, combine potatoes, 1½ teaspoons of oil, half the chili powder, salt, and pepper. Toss until well coated.

4. Transfer to the baking sheet in a single layer. Arrange the bell peppers on the tray. Bake for 30 minutes.

5. Remove and allow to cool, cutting the peppers into strips.

6. Toast the almonds over medium heat for 3 minutes.

7. Add in the remainder of the oil, chili, salt and pepper, sugar, and zest. Cook for 1 minute, stirring occasionally.

8. Divide the cooked quinoa among 4 bowls and top evenly with kale and potato mixture.

9. Share the almonds and avocado between the bowls.

10. Serve.

Calories: 591 kcal | Fat: 32 g | Protein: 16 g | Carbohydrates: 67 g

Mushroom-Asparagus Bowl

Buying pre-cooked farro will save you some time; however, cooking it yourself isn't that hard. It just takes a little while. You can add a handful of crisped tofu for a little extra body. If you are not following a fully vegetarian or vegan approach to the plant-based diet, you can add about a ¼ cup of shredded chicken breast per serving.

This recipe makes 4 servings.

What you need:

- 2 tablespoons olive oil
- 3 cup shiitake mushrooms, sliced
- 1 clove garlic, crushed
- 2 small sweet red onions, thinly sliced
- 1½ cups asparagus, cut into thirds
- 4 cups farro, cooked
- 1 tablespoon vegan butter
- 1 teaspoon lemon zest

- 2 tablespoons lemon juice
- ⅓ cup spring onions, cut into thirds
- ¼ cup toasted almonds
- ¼ cup shredded vegan cheese
- 2 tablespoons fresh dill

What to do:

1. In a large frying pan, heat the oil and cook the mushrooms until their liquid has evaporated.
2. Add garlic and cook until fragrant. Remove from the pan and set aside.
3. Return the pan to the stove and heat 2 tablespoons of oil, adding the asparagus, spring onions, and red onions, cooking until just soft.
4. Remove from the pan and set aside.
5. Place the farro in a large bowl. Stir in the butter, zest, and lemon juice until thoroughly incorporated.
6. Divide among 4 bowls, topping evenly with the mushrooms and vegetable mixtures.

7. Sprinkle almonds and cheese before serving.

Calories: 267 kcal | Fat: 13 g | Protein: 11 g | Carbohydrates: 38 g

Veggie Bolognese

This fragrant, vegan version of Bolognese will make you switch this out for every meal. Add an extra sprinkling of vegan cheese when serving for a little bit of extra indulgence.

This recipe makes 4 servings.

What you need:

- 2 tablespoons olive oil
- 2 teaspoons fennel seed
- 2 whole bay leaves
- 1 teaspoon cayenne pepper
- 1 cup dried porcini mushrooms (soaked in 1½ cups water)
- 3 cups shiitake mushrooms, sliced

- 1 cup onion
- 1 cup carrots, chopped
- ½ cup celery, chopped
- 1½ cup tempeh, crumbled
- 1 teaspoon salt
- 1 teaspoon pepper
- 3½ cups whole peeled tomatoes (1 large can)
- 5 cloves garlic, crushed
- 1 cup coconut milk
- ½ dry red wine
- 2 tablespoons oregano and basil, freshly chopped
- ½ vegan cheese, shredded
- 1 teaspoon brown sugar
- 1 tablespoon began butter
- Dried spaghetti for 4 servings

What to do:

1. In a small pan over medium heat, toast the

fennel, cayenne pepper, and bay leaves until fragrant.

2. Allow to cool before adding to a grinder, and pulverizing to a fine powder. Set aside.

3. Save ½ cup of the mushroom water and drain the rest, chopping the porcini mushrooms. Add to a food processor, along with the onions, carrots, and celery. Pulse until finely chopped.

4. In a large deep cooking pot, heat the oil over medium heat and add the tempeh, cooking for 5 minutes.

5. Add the fresh mushrooms with a pinch of salt and pepper, cooking 5 more minutes.

6. Finally, add in the porcini mixture, garlic, and spices, cooking a further 5 minutes, mixing occasionally.

7. Chop or pulse the tomatoes until fine, stirring into the mushroom mixture. Add in the milk, wine, herbs, sugar, zest, and mushroom water.

8. Reduce the heat, cover partially with a lid, and allow to simmer for an hour.

9. Stir in the cheese before serving.

10. Cook spaghetti per instructions, and add the butter, carefully tossing to coat.

11. Divide and serve with the Bolognese.

Calories: 353 kcal | Fat: 10 g | Protein: 16 g | Carbohydrates: 53 g

Sweet Potato and Lentil Curry

The potatoes add a delicious, filling element to this flavorsome curry.

This recipe makes 8 servings.

What you need:

- 4 cups sweet potato, peeled, cubed
- 3 cups water, divided
- 2 cups red lentils
- 2 cups vegetable stock
- ¾ cup white onion, chopped
- ½ cup red onion, sliced

- 3 tablespoons red curry paste
- 2 teaspoons masala
- 2 teaspoons turmeric powder
- 2 teaspoons grated ginger
- 2 teaspoons brown sugar
- ½ teaspoon salt and pepper
- 3 cloves garlic, crushed
- ¾ cup tomato paste (or 1 can)
- 1 cup coconut milk
- ½ cup apple cider vinegar
- 4 cups brown rice, cooked

What to do:

1. In a 6-quart slow cooker or a large pot, add water, stock, potato, lentil, white onion, curry and tomato paste, ginger, garlic, and spices, stirring well to combine. (It is ideal to use a slow cooker. If you use a pot, you will need to keep an eye on it and adjust with water as it evaporates.)

2. Cook for 8 hours or until the ingredients are well cooked.

3. When ready, remove from heat. Add in the coconut milk, and let stand for 5 minutes.

4. In a microwave-safe bowl, combine ½ cup of water, 2 teaspoons sugar, and vinegar.

5. Microwave on high for 2 minutes, stirring at intervals.

6. When the liquid starts to boil, remove and add the red onion to the mixture and allow to sit for 20–30 minutes.

To serve:

1. Place ½ cup of rice in each of 8 shallow bowls, topping each serving with 1¼ cups of the lentil and potato mixture.

2. Drain the red onions and spoon evenly onto each serving.

Calories: 395 kcal | Fat: 3 g | Protein: 17 g | Carbohydrates: 75 g

Orange-Tofu Stir-Fry

This is a light, citrusy stir-fry, perfect hot or cold.

This recipe makes 4 servings.

What you need:

- ¼ cup canola oil, divided
- 5 tablespoons cornstarch, divided
- 2–3 cups firm tofu, drained thoroughly and cubed
- ½ cup fresh orange juice
- 1 cup onion
- 1 cup green and red bell pepper, sliced thinly
- 2 cloves garlic, thinly sliced
- ½ teaspoon orange zest
- ½ teaspoon crushed red pepper
- 3 tablespoons soy sauce
- 1 tablespoon rice vinegar
- 1 teaspoon brown sugar

- ½ teaspoon salt
- ½ teaspoon pepper
- 2 cups brown rice, cooked

What to do:

1. Heat half of the oil in a skillet over medium-high heat.
2. In a bowl, toss the tofu with 4 tablespoons of cornstarch until well coated.
3. Add to the heated oil, cooking until the tofu is crispy and golden brown.
4. Remove from heat and drain on a paper towel.
5. In a separate bowl, combine the remaining cornstarch and orange juice. Whisk until there are no more clumps.
6. Heat another pan on medium heat, adding the onions and peppers, cooking for 5 minutes.
7. Add garlic, zest, and crushed red pepper, stirring until well combined and fragrant.
8. Add the orange juice mixture, soy, vinegar,

sugar, and salt. Bring to a boil.

9. Stir in the tofu just before serving.

10. To serve, divide the rice between 4 plates, topping each with about ¾ cup of the tofu mixture.

Calories: 488 kcal | Fat: 22 g | Protein: 17 g | Carbohydrates: 59 g

Lentil-Tahini Burger

The trick to binding this savory lentil burger together is tahini. This recipe is definitely a must if you are looking for an egg-free patty to add to your regular meals. The recipe goes a lot quicker if you are able to find steamed, vacuum-packed lentils. Not only do they provide the best texture, but it removes the extra hassle of cooking them up yourself. If you cannot find these, make you own. Simmer ½ cup of brown lentils in 4 cups of water for 20 minutes and drain well. Adding in the handful of pickled cabbage lends and extra zingy kick that perfectly balances out this earthy treat.

This recipe makes 4 patties.

What you need:

- 2 cups red cabbage, finely shredded
- 3 tablespoons red wine vinegar
- ½ teaspoon salt
- 1 teaspoon sesame seeds
- 4 tablespoons olive oil
- ½ cup onion, chopped
- ¼ cup tahini
- ½ teaspoon ground cumin
- ½ teaspoon black pepper
- 1⅓ cups lentils, cooked
- ½ cup carrot, grated
- 3 tablespoons soy yogurt
- ¼ cup chopped cilantro
- 2 teaspoons fresh lemon juice
- ½ small garlic clove, grated
- 2 teaspoons water

- 4 whole-wheat hamburger buns, toasted

What to do:

1. In a small bowl, combine cabbage, vinegar, and salt. Allow to stand 20 minutes before draining.

2. Mix in the sesame seeds.

3. In a large skillet over medium heat, add 3 tablespoons oil and cook the onion for 3 minutes.

4. In a food processor (or with a small hand chopper/grinder), coarsely chop 2 tablespoons tahini, cumin, pepper, and lentils.

5. Add to the cooked lentils in a separate bowl, mixing well with onions, carrots, and cilantro. Divide mixture and shape into 4 patties.

6. Heat remaining tablespoons oil in pan.

7. Cook the patties 4 minutes each side until a slightly crispy edge is formed.

8. To make the yogurt sauce, combine remaining 2 tablespoons tahini, yogurt, juice, and garlic in a bowl and mix well.

9. Stir in the water, a little at a time, until a smooth,

creamy sauce is formed (you can add more or less for your own desired consistency).

10. To serve, spread the yogurt mixture over the bottom halves of the buns. Top with a warm patty. Scoop cabbage over the patty and top with the bun.

Calories: 349 kcal | Fat: 15.5 g | Protein: 13 g | Carbohydrates: 44 g

Chickpea and Bulgur Wheat Burgers

You do not need to mash the chickpeas completely smooth, as the lumps add a little extra texture to these burger patties. Be careful as the raw chickpea mixture is delicate. It will firm up as it cooks, but be gentle when turning over in the pan so that they do not fall apart. Pre-cooking bulgur and saving it for later will make this recipe really quick and easy to make.

This recipe makes 4 patties.

What you need:

- ¾ cup water

- 1⅓ cup bulgur, cooked
- 2 cups chickpeas, cooked (or 1 can)
- ⅔ cup green onion, chopped
- 1 teaspoon ground cumin
- 1 teaspoon paprika
- 1 teaspoon salt
- ½ cup unsweetened applesauce (or two eggs, if not vegan)
- 1 tablespoon olive oil
- 1 large ripe avocado
- 1 clove garlic, crushed
- 4 whole-wheat hamburger buns

What to do:

1. Place drained chickpeas in a large bowl and mash until almost smooth.
2. Mix in spring onions, ground cumin, ¾ teaspoons salt, paprika, and applesauce.
3. Stir in the bulgur wheat and shape into 4 patties.

4. In a large skillet, heat the olive oil over medium heat and add the patties to the pan.

5. Cook carefully on each side until brown.

6. Combine avocado, the rest of the salt, and garlic in a bowl and mash together until smooth. Sprinkle a bit of lemon juice to keep from browning.

7. Divide and spread evenly between the buns and top with a patty.

8. You can add a slice of tomato and a shred of lettuce for a cool, crisp lunch burger.

Calories: 409 kcal | Fat: 13 g | Protein: 11 g | Carbohydrates: 56 g

Black Bean and Mushroom Burger

If you have a food processor, these burger patties will come together in no time. The mushrooms that give this burger its meaty texture is all thanks to the cremini mushrooms (also known as baby bellas). They have a much stronger, earthier taste than white button mushrooms. The accompanying avo mixture is great not just with burgers but also with sandwiches and breakfast toasts.

You can double the recipe of these burger patties and freeze them for later use. They will hold up to a month in the freezer.

This recipe makes 4 patties.

What you need:

- 1 tablespoon ground flaxseed
- 1 tablespoon Worcestershire sauce
- ½ teaspoon cumin
- ½ teaspoon pepper
- 3 cups cremini mushrooms
- 2 cups black beans, cooked (or one 15-ounce can)
- ¼ cup unsweetened applesauce
- 1 clove garlic
- ⅓ cup breadcrumbs
- 1 tablespoon olive oil

- 2 tablespoons vegan yogurt
- 2 tablespoons fresh lime juice
- 1 large avocado
- 2 tablespoons water
- 4 whole-wheat hamburger buns, toasted
- ½ cup red cabbage, shredded

What to do:

1. In a food processor, add the flaxseed, Worcestershire sauce, a pinch of salt, cumin, pepper, mushrooms, half of the beans, applesauce, and garlic.

2. Pulse until just smooth.

3. Stir in the remaining beans and the breadcrumbs. The mixture should be firm but not completely dry. Divide into 4 to make the patties.

4. Heat the oil on medium heat, cooking the patties until browned (approximately 3 minutes per side).

5. Combine ¼ teaspoons salt, juice, and avocado in a bowl, mashing together with a fork.

6. Mix in the yogurt until smooth.

7. Add water to adjust the consistency.

8. Add patties to buns and top with avocado-yogurt mixture and cabbage.

9. Serve.

Calories: 350 kcal | Fat: 13 g | Protein: 14 g | Carbohydrates: 48 g

Mushroom and Zucchini Bowl

This recipe makes 2 servings.

What you need:

- 1 medium-sized zucchini
- ½ teaspoon salt
- ½ teaspoon pepper
- 2 tablespoons olive oil
- 1 cup yellow onion, chopped
- 1 tablespoon chopped garlic

- 1 tablespoon tomato paste
- 2–3 cups cremini mushrooms, sliced
- 1 can (approx. 28 ounces) tomatoes, fire-roasted, undrained
- 1 teaspoon black pepper
- 3 cups baby spinach
- ½ cup vegan ricotta (see lasagna recipe)
- ¾ cup vegan cheese, shredded
- ¼ cup fresh basil

What to do:

1. Using a vegetable peeler, "shave" zucchini into thin strips. Sprinkle with some salt and set aside.
2. In a deep cooking pot, heat the oil and cook the onion and garlic.
3. Add mushrooms and cook until browned.
4. Stir in tomato paste until mixed well.
5. Add in the tomatoes, pepper, and ½ teaspoons salt. Bring to a light simmer and stir frequently.

Allow the liquid to reduce slightly.

6. Add in spinach, cover, and remove from heat.

7. Mix in the zucchini after 3 minutes.

8. In a microwave-safe bowl, combine the ricotta and shredded cheese melt.

9. Stir frequently until melted.

10. Spoon over the zucchini mixture and sprinkle with basil.

Calories: 276 kcal | Fat: 13 g | Protein: 16 g | Carbohydrates: 26 g

Veggie Meatloaf

This recipe makes 6 servings.

What you need:

- 1 large red bell pepper
- 1 large green bell pepper
- 3 cups cremini mushrooms, coarsely chopped
- 1 tablespoon olive oil
- 1 cup asparagus, cut into thirds

- ½ cup red onion, chopped
- 1 cup breadcrumbs
- 1 cup walnuts, chopped
- 2 tablespoons fresh basil, finely chopped
- 1 tablespoon tomato puree
- 1 teaspoon Dijon mustard
- ½ teaspoon salt
- ½ teaspoon pepper
- ½ cup vegan cheese, grated
- ½ cup unsweetened applesauce (you can also use an egg replacer for two eggs, if you wish)

For the topping:

- 2 tablespoons ketchup
- 1 tablespoon vegetable stock
- ¼ teaspoon Dijon mustard

What to do:

1. Preheat oven to 400 degrees Fahrenheit.

2. Halve the bell peppers lengthwise, discarding seeds and membranes.

3. Place pepper halves, skin up, on a prepared baking sheet.

4. Press down firmly and bake for 12–15 minutes or until the peppers are blackened.

5. Remove from the oven and set aside to cool.

6. Peel and finely chop the peppers, placing them in a bowl and set aside.

7. Reduce oven temperature to 350 degrees Fahrenheit.

8. Add mushrooms in a food processor and pulse until finely chopped.

9. Transfer the chopped mushrooms to a bowl.

10. Heat the oil in a large skillet over medium-high heat and cook the mushrooms for about 15 minutes, allowing their liquid to evaporate, stirring occasionally.

11. Transfer mushrooms to the bowl with the bell pepper.

12. Add asparagus and onion to pan and cook until just tender.

13. Add onion mixture to mushroom mixture.

14. Lay breadcrumbs in an even layer on a baking sheet and bake for 10 minutes.

15. Add breadcrumbs and the rest of the ingredients together, mixing well.

16. Spoon the mixture into prepared loaf pan and press down gently to even out.

17. Bake for 45 minutes.

To prepare the topping:

1. Combine the topping ingredients together in a small bowl. Mix well.

2. Using a pastry brush, brush mixture over the slightly cooled meatloaf.

3. Bake an additional 10 minutes.

4. Remove from the oven and allow to sit 10 minutes.

5. Slice into 6 even slices.

Calories: 338 kcal | Fat: 21.2 g | Protein: 17.5 g | Carbohydrates: 22.6 g

Butternut Chickpea Stew

This is a hearty stew that is perfect, especially as a wintertime meal.

This recipe makes 4 servings.

What you need:

- 1½ tablespoons olive oil
- 1½ cups onion, chopped
- 2 cloves garlic, minced
- ½ teaspoon salt
- ½ teaspoon paprika
- ½ teaspoon cumin
- ¼ teaspoon ground ginger
- ¼ teaspoon cinnamon
- ¼ teaspoon black pepper

- 1 tablespoon tomato paste
- 3 cups butternut squash, diced and peeled
- 2 cups chickpeas
- 2 cups diced tomatoes (approx. 1 can or 15 ounces)
- 1½ cups vegetable stock
- 1½ cups quinoa, cooked
- 2 cups arugula
- ¼ cup vegan yogurt

What to do:

1. Heat oil in a large cooking pot over medium-high heat and add the onion and garlic.
2. Cook until soft and fragrant.
3. Stir in the spices and cook 1 minute.
4. Stir in tomato paste and cook.
5. Add squash and chickpeas, cooking for a further 2 minutes.
6. Add in tomatoes and stock, and bring to a boil.

7. Reduce to a simmer and cook 20 minutes.

8. Divide the quinoa among 4 bowls and top evenly with squash mixture, arugula, and yogurt.

Calories: 413 kcal | Fat: 9 g | Protein: 17 g | Carbohydrates: 69 g

Cauli-Korma

This dish is delicious served on steamed rice. The almonds add a wonderful crunch to this flavorful dish. You can substitute the almonds for cashews for a slightly softer crunch but still just as tasty.

This recipe makes 6 servings.

What you need:

- 1 tablespoon olive oil
- ⅓ cup onion, chopped
- ½ cup carrot, finely chopped
- 2 teaspoons curry powder
- ½ teaspoon salt

- ½ teaspoon pepper
- ½ teaspoon ginger
- ¼ teaspoon garam masala
- 2 cloves garlic, minced
- 3–4 cups cauliflower florets
- 2½ cups vegetable stock
- 1 cup vegan yogurt
- ¾ cup green peas, cooked and drained
- 2½ cup brown rice, cooked
- ½ cup fresh cilantro leaves
- ½ cup roasted almonds, chopped

What to do:

1. Over a medium, add oil in a pan.
2. Add onions and carrots and cook 2 minutes or until onion is translucent.
3. Add in curry powder and other spices.
4. Cook until fragrant.

5. Stir in cauliflower, cooking for 5 minutes, stirring occasionally.

6. Add the stock and bring to a light simmer.

7. Cover and cook until cauliflower is tender.

8. Remove from heat and set aside, keeping the juices in a small bowl.

9. Add yogurt to ½ cup of this liquid, and stir until smooth.

10. Stir mixture into cauliflower and add peas.

11. Combine well.

12. Transfer ⅔ cup of rice in each of the 6 bowls.

13. Top each serving with 1 cup cauliflower mixture.

14. Evenly divide cilantro and almonds.

Calories: 270 kcal | Fat: 12 g | Protein: 9 g | Carbohydrates: 33 g

Snacks and Appetizers

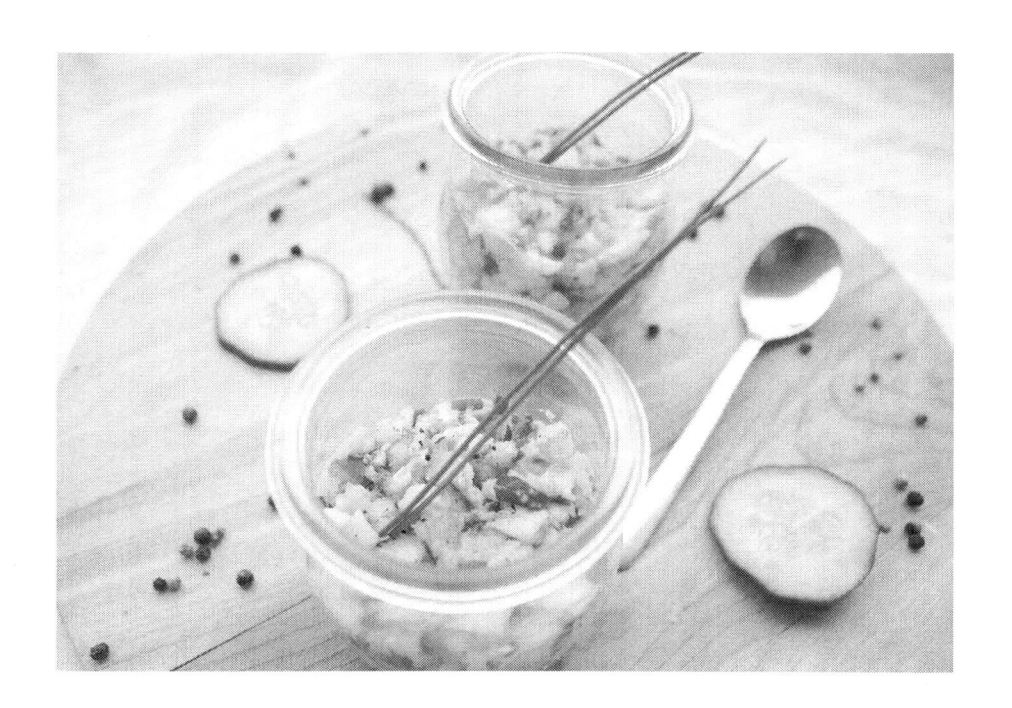

Chocolate Chip Granola Bars

This recipe is a good way to make use of the leftover almond pulp, or alternatively, you can just use fine, blanched almond flour. You can snack on these at breakfast, lunch, or as a light dessert to tide you over until your next meal.

If you are using homemade almond pulp, make sure to squeeze out the excess moisture really well. Layer on a paper towel and store in the fridge overnight as this helps to dry it out a little more.

Some recipes would require you to cook your pulp in a dehydrator to reach that "flour" texture. You do not need to use one. It simply means your bars will have a little more moisture and will need to be baked a little bit longer. You also do not want it too wet. Do not use it immediately after making your almond milk because it could make the bars too wet, and the result would not be as good. They are delicious either way, whether you use pulp or flour.

This recipe makes 8 bars.

What you need:

- ½ cup + 2 tablespoons maple syrup, room temperature (you can use agave nectar as well)
- ¼ cup ground flaxseed
- 1 cup almond pulp or blanched almond flour
- 1 cup whole rolled oats (do not use instant or quick oats)
- 2 teaspoons ground cinnamon

- ½ teaspoon fine sea salt

- 1/2 cup mini dairy-free chocolate chips (or a dairy-free bar, chopped into small pieces)

- ½ cup almond butter

- 2 teaspoons vanilla extract

What to do:

1. Preheat an oven to 350 degrees Fahrenheit.

2. Line a 9×5-inch loaf pan with parchment paper. (It is preferred that you do not use a different sized pan, as this will affect how these bars will turn out. They need to be just the right size and thickness for the best results.)

3. Mix the syrup and flaxseed in a small bowl, whisking with a fork until well combined.

4. Set aside. (Skipping this step will make your bars fall apart and not keep their shape. This is what binds them together like normal eggs would.)

5. In a separate bowl, add the almond pulp (or almond flour), oats, cinnamon, and salt. Mix well.

6. Stir in the chocolate chips.

7. When the syrup mixture has set for at least 10 minutes, combine with the almond butter and vanilla until super smooth.

8. Pour over the dry ingredients and stir until very sticky and absorbed.

9. Add the dough to the loaf pan and spread out evenly and flat with a rubber spatula.

10. Important: For dough using almond pulp, bake for 30–35 minutes (until the tops are firm and dark golden brown).

11. For dough using almond flour, bake for 25–30 minutes (until the tops are firm and dark golden brown).

12. Allow to cool for at least 1 hour before cutting to prevent them from crumbling apart.

13. You can melt some chocolate to drizzle over the tops for added chocolaty sweetness.

14. Wrap each individually in plastic wrap and store in the fridge.

Sandwiches with Hummus Spread

This spread is delicious as a lunchbox filler or an easy-to-assemble at-home snack or light meal.

This recipe makes 1 sandwich.

What you need:

- 2 slices of bread of choice (you can use some of the breads you have baked using these recipes or your favorite store-bought)
- 3–4 tablespoons hummus (homemade version below)
- Vegetables of choice, sliced thinly: beet, tomato, carrot, yellow bell pepper, lettuce, baby greens, and cucumber

What to do:

1. Toast your slices of bread.
2. Spread the hummus evenly onto one side of each slice.
3. Layer your vegetables on one side of the sandwich.

4. For a nice "rainbow" effect, layer them according to color—ROYGBIV (red, orange, yellow, green, blue, indigo, violet).

5. Close the sandwich by placing the other slice of bread on top.

6. You can wrap these in parchment paper and pop into a lunchbox for later if you are not going to be eating these rights away.

Coconut Bacon

Sprinkle on burgers, salads, or just nibble on as a small snack!

What you need:

- 3½ cups coconut flakes, unsweetened
- 2 tablespoons liquid smoke
- 1 tablespoon liquid aminos or soy sauce
- 1 tablespoon maple syrup
- 1 tablespoon water
- 1 teaspoon smoked paprika (optional)

What to do:

1. Preheat oven to 325 degrees Fahrenheit.
2. Prepare a baking tray with parchment paper.
3. In a large bowl, combine liquid smoke, aminos, maple syrup, and water and mix together.
4. Add in flaked coconut using a wooden spoon to gently toss the coconut in the liquid mixture.
5. Sprinkle paprika over and toss.
6. Once the coconut is evenly coated, pour onto the prepared baking sheet.
7. Bake for 20–25 minutes.
8. Use a spatula to flip the coconut every 5 minutes to cook it evenly.
9. Keep a constant eye on this as it will burn. Flip frequently.
10. Coconut "bacon" can be stored in a sealed ziplock bag or airtight container for up to a month.

Black Bean Tostada

This is beans and salsa in a crisp shell—quick and easy.

This recipe makes 6 servings.

What you need:

- 1 can refried black beans (approx. 15 oz.)
- ½ cup salsa (you can make it yourself or buy premade from the supermarket)
- 4 tablespoons olive oil
- 2 tablespoons red wine vinegar
- 1 teaspoon oregano
- ½ teaspoon salt and pepper
- 1½ cups shredded cabbage
- 1 cup radishes, thinly sliced
- 1 cup baby tomatoes, halves
- ½ cup red onion, thinly sliced
- 6 corn tostada shells
- 1½ cups vegan cheese (the extra melty kind)

- Torn fresh cilantro for sprinkling

What to do:

1. In a small saucepan, heat a splash of oil and add the beans and salsa.
2. Cook over medium heat, stirring often for about 5 minutes.
3. Remove from heat, and cover to keep warm.
4. In a large bowl, whisk together oil, vinegar, oregano, salt, and pepper until well combined.
5. Add cabbage, radishes, tomatoes, and onions and toss to combine.
6. Allow to stand 5 minutes to absorb the flavor.
7. Fill each tostada shell with approximately ⅓ cup bean mixture and 1 cup cabbage mixture.
8. Divide the cheese between the shells and top with a sprinkling of cilantro.

Calories: 324 kcal | Fat: 20 g | Protein: 12 g | Carbohydrate: 27 g

Desserts

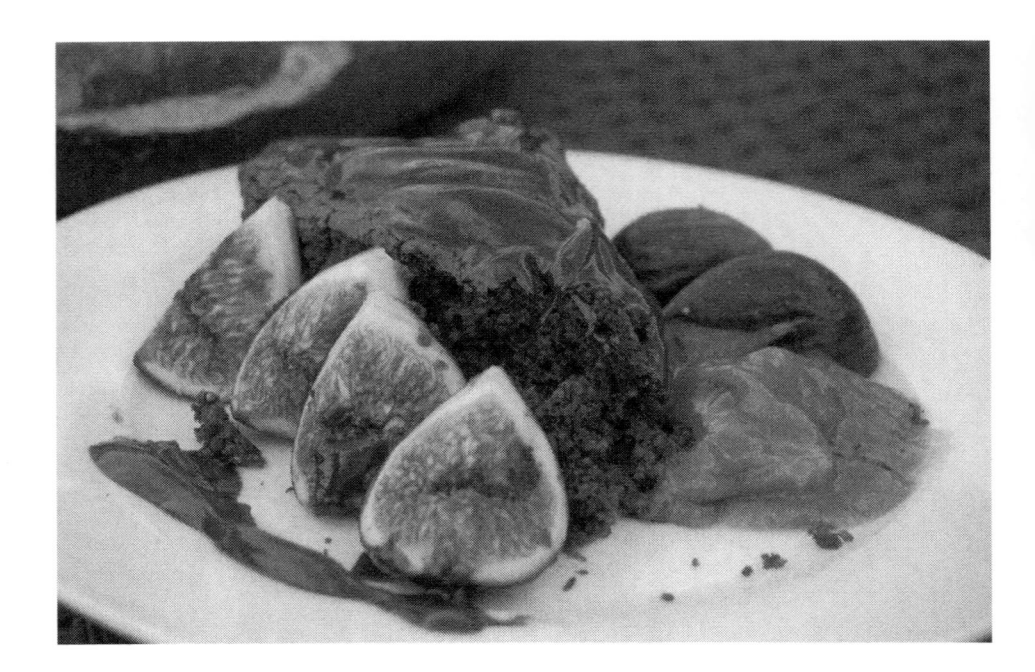

Ginger Cookies

These ginger cookies are different from the classic in the fact that the oil is replaced with coconut butter instead. It gives them an amazing new level of flavor, sweetness, and texture.

They do not taste like coconut, so there will be no

excuse to not indulge in these once in a while. The key here is to use good-quality coconut butter. Ensure the butter is properly melted when measuring out. You can pop it in the microwave for a few seconds and stir frequently do distribute the clumps for better melting.

These vegan-friendly cookies are sweet, spicy, and perfectly buttery.

A little note: To make these gluten-free, substitute with superfine oat flour. Adjust the quantity to 1¾ cup + 2 tablespoons of oat flour. All the other ingredients are still the same, and you will bake for the same amount of time.

Before adding the coconut butter, make sure the butter is completely liquid before measuring, so the right amount is added and the cookies turn out moist. The coconut butter will separate during storage, so heat the jar a little and mix with a spoon. Heat a few more seconds in the microwave, stirring until it is smooth and runny. Then measure. This will ensure accurate results.

This recipe makes 18 cookies.

What you need:

- 1½ cups spelt flour
- ½ teaspoon baking soda
- 2 teaspoons ground cinnamon
- 1½ teaspoons ground allspice
- 1½ tablespoons ground ginger
- ½ teaspoon sea salt
- ½ cup + 2 tablespoons maple syrup, at room temperature
- 3 tablespoons molasses (do not use blackstrap molasses)
- ½ cup + 2 tablespoons melted coconut butter (not coconut oil, which is completely different)
- Optional: some white icing sugar for sprinkling

What to do:

1. Preheat oven to 350 degrees Fahrenheit.
2. Prepare two baking sheets with parchment paper and set aside.
3. Add the flour, baking soda, cinnamon, allspice,

ginger, and salt to a large bowl and combine well.

4. Make a well in the middle of the dry ingredients, and add the syrup, molasses, and the liquid coconut butter.

5. Mix the batter together until just combined. It should form into a sticky, thick batter (the oat flour version will pull away from the sides and form a ball instead).

6. Scoop 1½ tablespoons to form dough balls.

7. Place on the pans approximately 3 inches apart (do not add more than 9 balls to each pan) and flatten ¼ inch thick.

8. Sprinkle icing sugar on top for extra sweetness and crunch, if desired.

9. Bake for 8 minutes (one pan at a time). They will spread out a little and puff up. Do not bake longer than 10 minutes as they will dry out.

10. They should be firm and golden on the bottoms. Remove from the oven and allow to cool for 10 minutes.

11. Transfer to a cooling rack and store in an airtight container.

Calories: 144.2 kcal | Fat: 5.6 g | Protein: 1.9 g | Carbohydrates: 21.2 g

Choc-Mint Ice Cream

Note: To make this a starch-free version, just add a ¼ cup of raw cashews or almonds with the other ingredients to a blender. You can soak the nuts beforehand for a few hours to soften and make the blending process easier, drain thoroughly before continuing.

What you need:

- 2 cups coconut milk, full fat
- 1 cup almond milk
- ¼ cup + 2 tablespoons sugar
- ½ cup sweet potato, cooked and mashed
- 1 teaspoon vanilla extract
- ¼ cup cocoa powder

- 2 tablespoons crushed peppermint candy (or 1–2 teaspoons peppermint essence)
- 1 tablespoon cornstarch
- ¼ teaspoon sea salt

What to do:

1. Shake the cans of coconut milk well before decanting.
2. In a blender, add the potato, milk, and cocoa powder. Pulse until creamy.
3. Transfer the blended mixture in a small deep cooking pot. Add the sugar, cornstarch, salt, and half the peppermint candy (or essence). Whisk well.
4. Turn the heat to medium and allow to simmer until the mixture thickens.
5. Continue whisking as it cooks.
6. Remove from the heat and whisk in the vanilla.
7. Transfer the mixture into an airtight plastic container and chill (skip to the end of the recipe for a machine-free method).

8. Make sure it has completely cooled and chilled at least 2 hours before pouring into your ice-cream maker. If it is too hot, it will take ages to make. Let the machine do its thing for approximately 15 minutes. (Note: If you do not have an ice-cream maker, you could make these as popsicles as well. Just pour into molds and freeze overnight.)

9. Add in the remaining peppermint and allow to churn for a further minute.

10. Serve.

Machine-free:

1. Use the freezer as follows: After transferring the ice cream to the airtight container, add a layer of plastic wrap, pressing it down to make contact with the ice cream. This will eliminate the ice crystal formation.

2. Pop your container into the freezer and leave overnight.

3. Note: You can also stir the mixture every few hours to assist the process. It will help to avoid the ice crystals that will affect the texture.

Remember to reseal with plastic wrap as well.

Calories: 155.7 kcal | Fat: 8.6 g | Carbohydrates: 17.7 | Protein: 2.25 g

Spicy Chocolate Fudge

You can omit the chili flakes to make simple chocolate fudge. These are beautiful with or without the kick, although this is for spicy lovers only. It is important that your liquids are at room temperature. This will keep the chocolate from hardening too soon.

This recipe makes 10 pieces.

What you need:

- ½ cup packed sweet potato, cooked and mashed
- 200 grams (7 ounces) 70% dark chocolate, finely chopped
- ¼ teaspoon salt
- ¼ cup maple syrup, room temperature
- 2 tablespoons plant milk of choice, room temperature

- ⅛ teaspoons ground chili pepper
- ¼ teaspoon cinnamon
- ½ teaspoon vanilla extract

What to do:

1. Add the potato to a food processor.
2. Finely chop the chocolate. Transfer it to a microwave-safe bowl and melt at an interval of 10–30-seconds, stirring frequently.
3. Add the salt to the chocolate and stir.
4. Add the chocolate to the food processor, scraping all of it out of the bowl using a rubber spatula. Whizz until smooth.
5. Add the syrup, milk, and spices. Whizz again for at least a minute until completely smooth, scraping the sides, adding in the vanilla as you go. (It is supposed to have a rich, dark chocolate taste, but feel free to adjust to your liking. Should you feel like a little more sweetness, add a tablespoon of fine sugar or similarly granulated sweetener. Do not add any more liquid!).

6. Line a loaf pan with a baking sheet.

7. Transfer the fudge to the pan and evenly spread out with a rubber spatula out to the corners.

8. For an extra spicy kick, sprinkle chili flakes over the top. For a sweeter nibble, add coconut sugar.

9. Cover with plastic wrap and allow to cool in the fridge to firm up for several hours or overnight before slicing.

10. Keep stored in the fridge.

Calories: 155.7 kcal | Fat: 8.6 g | Carbohydrates: 17.7 g | Protein: 2.25 g

Basic Vanilla Buttercream Frosting

Perfect buttercream is found in a delicate blend of shortening and butter. You can use this to cover cakes, cupcakes, and muffins. Add in some food coloring to mix up some pretty designs!

This recipe covers 14 cupcakes.

What you need:

- ½ cup vegan butter

- ½ cup Spectrum shortening (or a similar type if you cannot find it)

- 2½ cups powdered sugar

- 1 tablespoon coconut milk or milk of choice

- 1 teaspoon white vanilla powder for a white frosting or 1 teaspoon vanilla extract, which will tint it slightly

What to do:

1. Make sure that the vegan butter is left at room temperature so that it is soft and easy to blend.

2. Add the vegan butter and shortening to a stand mixer and beat on low until just blended (you can mix this with a wooden spoon, but it would take a bit longer).

3. Add the sugar a cup at a time being sure to blend fully before adding the next.

4. Add the milk and vanilla last and beat until light and fluffy.

5. Cover with plastic wrap to keep it moist until

ready to frost, or you may store it in the fridge until needed.

6. Set out an hour before use to soften for use.

Calories: 191 kcal | Protein: 7 g | Fat: 13.8 g | Carbohydrates: 18.4 g

Chocolate Frosting

Perfect buttercream is found in a delicate blend of shortening and butter. You can use this to cover cakes, cupcakes, and muffins. It is delicious and chocolatey! Just do not eat it straight from the bowl (yes, it is that delicious).

This frosting can be stored in the freezer up to 3 months. Thaw in the fridge overnight and then set out for an hour before use to soften. Once soft, beat lightly until fluffy and smooth before frosting a cake or piping onto cupcakes.

Double the frosting if you're making a two-layer cake.

Covers 14 cupcakes.

What you need:

- ½ cup vegan butter
- ½ cup Spectrum shortening (or a similar type if you cannot find it)
- 1½ cups powdered sugar
- ½ cup unsweetened cocoa powder
- 1 tablespoon almond milk or milk of choice
- ½ teaspoon vanilla extract

What to do:

1. Make sure that the vegan butter is left at room temperature so that it is soft and easy to blend.
2. Add the vegan butter and shortening to a stand mixer and beat on low until just blended (you can mix this with a wooden spoon, but it would take a bit longer).
3. Add the sugar a cup at a time. Make sure to blend fully before adding the next.
4. Add in the cocoa powder, and mix through.
5. Add the milk and vanilla last and beat until light and fluffy.

6. Store in the fridge if not using right away and let it come back to room temperature and soft before piping onto the cupcakes or cake.

Calories: 191 kcal | Protein: 7 g | Fat: 13.8 g | Carbohydrates: 18.4 g

Chocolate Cupcakes

These cupcakes are moist, chocolatey, and addictive. Frost or eat as is.

They freeze beautifully and are fantastic again once thawed. To thaw, simply place them out on the counter a few hours before serving. These cupcakes rise rather well, so it is important to divide the batter into 14 or 15 cupcakes.

This recipe makes 14 cupcakes.

What you need:

- 1 cup + 2 tablespoons all-purpose flour
- ¾ cup coconut sugar
- ¾ teaspoon baking soda

- ¼ + ⅛ teaspoons baking powder
- ½ teaspoon salt
- 1 cup unsweetened almond milk
- 3 ounce dairy-free dark chocolate chips
- 4½ tablespoons maple syrup
- 6 tablespoons unsweetened cocoa powder
- 1½ teaspoons ground dried espresso

What to do:

1. Preheat the oven to 350 degrees Fahrenheit.
2. Prepare two muffin tins, either with a cooking spray or with liners.
3. In a medium-sized bowl, add the flour, sugar, baking powder, baking soda, and salt, combining until properly mixed and lump-free.
4. In a separate, microwave-safe bowl, add the almond milk and chocolate chips.
5. Microwave intermittently for 30–45 seconds, stirring until the chocolate is melted and smooth.

6. Whisk in the syrup, cocoa powder, and espresso powder (if using) until smooth.

7. Slowly add the dry ingredients to the chocolate, stirring gently.

8. Once smooth, divide the batter into the muffin tins. Do not fill more than half per muffin hole.

9. Bake for 15–20 minutes (stick a toothpick in the center and remove from the oven when the toothpick comes out clean). Be careful not to over-bake as they will dry out.

10. Let the cupcakes cool completely before frosting.

Calories: 265 kcal | Protein: 5 g | Fat: 10.8 g | Carbohydrates: 38.4 g

Cinnamon Rolls

Coconut milk, mashed potatoes, and roasted walnut butter are used to replace the copious amounts of butter used in traditional cinnamon rolls.

Cook the Yukon Gold potatoes with the skin on,

wrapped in a damp paper towel in a microwave until soft and squishy (approximately 3–5 minutes). If you do not have a microwave, bake it in the oven. This will take much longer, but it is preferable over boiling or steaming. You do not want the added moisture this brings as it will affect the way the buns rise and cook.

Make the walnut butter beforehand; you can store it in airtight jars and use as needed.

You can bake the rolls in two different ways. Baking them separately will yield a firmer, crispier edge to the rolls. They are easy to simply grab and eat, no need to separate them first. If you prefer much softer edges, as with the traditional kind, place them in two 9-inch round cake pans lined with parchment paper. Space them out slightly to allow them room to rise as they bake, letting them fluff up perfectly. This way will take longer to bake, so adjust the cooking time to 25 minutes or a bit longer, depending on your oven. They need to be a light golden brown on top.

This recipe makes about 10 rolls.

What you need:

For the dough:

- 3 cups all-purpose flour (the recipe works best with zero substitutions)
- 2¼ teaspoons instant yeast
- ¾ teaspoon salt
- 1 cup canned lite coconut milk (not full fat), room temperature, shaken before measured
- ¼ cup Yukon Gold potatoes, cooked, peeled, and mashed
- 3 tablespoons maple syrup
- ¼ cup roasted walnut butter (recipe is under sauces and condiments)
- 1½ teaspoons vanilla extract

For the filling:

- ½ cup coconut sugar
- 1½ tablespoons ground cinnamon
- ¼ cup roasted walnut butter

For the icing:

- 1 cup powdered sugar, sifted

- 2 tablespoons dairy-free, unsweetened yogurt
- ½ teaspoon lemon juice

What to do:

1. Add the flour, instant yeast, and salt to a deep bowl, and mix well.
2. Add the potato to a separate bowl. Add the milk, maple syrup, vanilla, and ¼ cup walnut butter (remember that there is another ¼ cup for the filling, so do not use this too).
3. Mix together quickly and transfer to a food processor. Whizz until perfectly smooth and liquidy.
4. Pour this mixture over the dry ingredients using a rubber spatula to get as much of the liquid as possible.
5. Stir a couple of minutes until it comes together into a roughly formed dough. It will seem dry at first, but do not add any more liquid. Stir until mostly combined and sprinkle flour on your work surface.

6. Scrape the dough out and knead. Do not overwork as it can make for tough rolls. It should not be sticky anymore but just easy to work with.

7. Add the dough to a bowl and cover with plastic wrap. Spray it with non-stick spray if it's a short or shallow bowl; otherwise, the dough will stick.

8. Allow to rise for 45 minutes to an hour. It should have doubled in size, so keep an eye on how it rises, as the environment will affect the time.

9. Preheat the oven to 350 degrees Fahrenheit and line a baking sheet with parchment paper.

10. When ready, scrape the dough back onto the lightly floured work surface.

11. Use a rolling pin to gently roll out into a rectangular shape, approximately 10½ inches wide by 16 inches long and ¼ inch thick.

12. Use a pastry brush to lightly brush on coconut milk in a thin layer. This will help the cinnamon-sugar mixture to adhere and add a little bit more moisture.

13. In another small bowl, combine the

cinnamon, coconut sugar, and the remaining walnut butter. Mix together well; it will be moist and crumbly.

14. Sprinkle this mixture evenly over the dough. Leave a ½-inch border along the edge.

15. Start with the longer end of the dough and gently roll it into a log. Be sure to roll it as tight as possible to eliminate the gaps.

16. Trim off the ends about 1–2 inches.

17. Using a very sharp knife, gently cut into rolls, approximately, 1½ inches thick. The dough should be soft but slices fairly easily. Be careful not to squash them down as you slice. Coat your knife lightly in flour between each slice as this will keep the knife from sticking and warping the rolls as you slice.

18. Carefully lay each roll onto the prepared baking tray, spaced at least 2 inches apart.

19. Bake for 15–20 minutes or until golden brown.

20. In a smaller bowl, add the icing ingredients

and mix until it is well blended and moist. Whisk until completely smooth and sugar is dissolved. Do not add any more liquid as this will come together as long as you keep whisking.

21. Remove the rolls from the oven and allow to rest 5–10 minutes.

22. Add a spoonful of icing on the center of each roll and spread around to let it drizzle down the sides.

23. Serve warm.

24. Store extra rolls in an airtight container at room temperature.

25. Reheat in the microwave for about 10–15 seconds.

26. You can make the dough ahead of time and store in the fridge or freezer. Remove from the freezer and place in the fridge overnight to defrost. Remove and set at room temperature for at least an hour before using. Cold dough will not rise or bake very well if cold.

Calories: 307 kcal | Protein: 5 g | Fat: 9.8 g |

Carbohydrates: 60.4 g

Peppermint Strawberry Cheesecake

This recipe makes approximately 8 slices.

What you need:

For the crust:

- 3½ cups almonds, slivered
- ¼ cup maple syrup
- 1 teaspoon vanilla extract

For the filling:

- 2½ cups whole cashews
- ½ cup maple syrup
- 3 cups strawberries
- ¼ cup lemon juice
- 1 teaspoon vanilla extract
- ⅛ teaspoons peppermint oil
- 1 cup water or plant milk

- ¼ teaspoon sea salt

What to do:

1. First, prepare the crust. Add the almonds to a food processor and pulse until fine.

2. Add the syrup and vanilla and pulse until well combined. It should clump together and stay together well.

3. Grease a springform pan and add the crust to the pan pressing down flat and evenly. If you use a different pan, line it with parchment paper to keep it from sticking to the pan.

4. In a food processor or high-powered blender, add all the filling ingredients and process until very smooth and creamy. When adding the peppermint oil, be sure to measure very carefully as it is strong. If you do not have a high-powered blender, soak the cashews overnight and drain before use.

5. Pour filling over the crust and place into the freezer overnight.

6. Cover with plastic wrap directly on top of the

cheesecake to prevent ice crystals.

7. Remove the cheesecake and set at room temperature for 15 minutes before serving to allow for an easy release from the pan. Do not let it sit out too long, or it will start to soften too much.

8. Garnish with thinly sliced strawberries and crushed peppermint, right before serving.

Calories: 177.7 kcal | Fat: 8.6 g | Carbohydrates: 20.7 g | Protein: 2.25 g

Sugar Cookies

Make these in batches and freeze the dough. The almond flour absolutely cannot be substituted out. There is no added oil, and any other flour will make it too dry.

This recipe makes 18 cookies.

What you need:

- 4½ tablespoons coconut sugar, powdered
- 1 cup + 2 tablespoons blanched almond flour

- 7 tablespoons potato starch (do not use potato flour; read the pack carefully)
- ¼ cup + 2 tablespoons white rice flour
- ½ teaspoon baking powder
- ½ teaspoon salt
- ½ cup maple syrup
- ¼ cup + 2 tablespoons cashew butter (use raw cashew butter, or make your own)
- 2½ teaspoons vanilla extract

What to do:

1. Preheat the oven to 350 degrees Fahrenheit.

2. Line two baking sheets with parchment paper and set aside (it is interesting to note that darker baking sheets will have the bottoms crisp up darker in the same amount of time compared to lighter-colored pans, which is what we want here).

3. Use a high-powered blender or coffee grinder to powder the coconut sugar. It needs to be fine in order to get the best texture.

4. Leave the lid on and allow the powder to settle before opening.

5. Add the sugar to a large bowl and mix in the dry ingredients one by one, giving it a stir between each.

6. In a separate bowl, add the syrup, cashew butter, and vanilla. It is better to use softer cashew butter to ensure the mixture blends and smooths down much better.

7. Pour this mixture over the dry ingredients.

8. Stir continuously as you add the liquid. The mixture should be firm once everything has been incorporated properly.

9. Divide the dough into 18 equal balls and pack onto the baking sheets.

10. Use a small piece of parchment paper to place over each ball, pressing flat into ¼ inch thickness.

11. Bake for 8–10 minutes. The tops should be puffy and the edges a slight crackled effect.

12. Allow to cool for 10 minutes before transferring to a wire rack.

13. Store in an airtight container.

Calories: 144.2 kcal | Fat: 5.6 g | Protein: 1.9 g | Carbohydrates: 21.2 g

Basic Sauces and Condiments

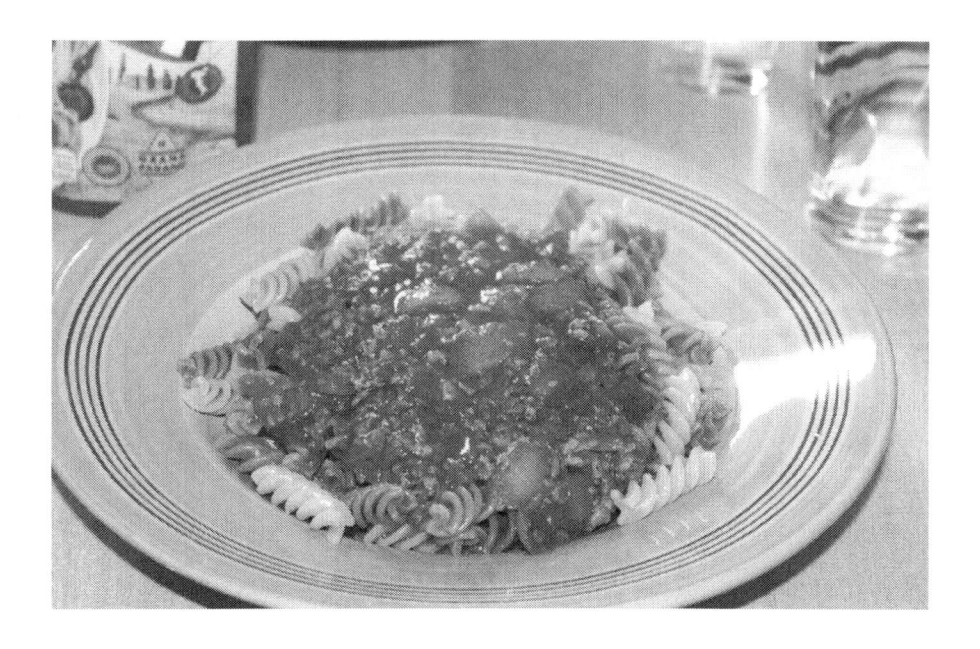

One of the ways to prepare your vegan cream sauce

depends on the base you are using. Many vegan sauces use either nuts or vegan butter as a base, such as a Béchamel sauce.

If it's a nut-based sauce, just soak the nuts overnight. Drain and toss them into a food processor to make them smooth and creamy (Kasee, 2018).

Cream Sauce

What you need:

- ½ cup gluten-free flour (can be any kind, such as chickpea, buckwheat, or millet)
- ½ cup nutritional yeast
- 1 teaspoon onion powder
- ½ teaspoon paprika
- ½ teaspoon mustard powder
- ½ teaspoon garlic powder
- ½ teaspoon cayenne pepper
- 2 cups nut milk of choice

- ¼ cup olive oil

- 1 teaspoon miso (or 2 teaspoons vegetable broth)

- Salt and pepper to taste

What to do:

1. In a medium-sized cooking pot, add the dry ingredients and slowly whisk in the nut milk, oil, and miso.

2. Turn the heat up to medium and simmer until the mixture thickens.

3. Continue stirring to ensure that the mixture does not burn.

4. Season with salt and pepper to taste.

Kale-and-Walnut Pesto

This kale-and-walnut pesto is simple and versatile, perfect for adding an extra zing to your favorite pasta or as a dip. If you do not have kale, any other leafy green vegetable will do. You can do half spinach and half arugula.

This recipe makes 1 cup of pesto.

What you need:

- ½ bunch kale, stems removed and chopped
- ½ cup walnuts, chopped
- 2 cloves garlic, crushed
- ¼ cup nutritional yeast
- ¼ cup lemon juice
- ¼ cup olive oil
- Salt and pepper to taste

What to do:

1. Bring a large pot of water to a boil, adding in the kale and ½ teaspoon of salt.
2. Cook until the leaves are soft, approximately 5 minutes.
3. Drain properly and transfer to a food processor.
4. Add the walnuts, garlic, nutritional yeast, olive oil, and lemon juice. Whizz until completely smooth.
5. Add salt and pepper to taste, adding in extra

lemon juice if you wish.

Spicy Vegan Dip

For this recipe, you will need to buy jackfruit in a can, most likely to be found in the international foods aisle or with the other Asian staples, such as rice noodles, coconut milk, and nori sheets. If you cannot find it, you may need to find an Asian grocery store or order through an online vendor.

Be sure to get the jackfruit in water (or brine if unavailable). Do not buy the kind that comes in syrup as these will be much too sweet and will be better in a dessert instead.

If you have never cooked with jackfruit before, be sure to check online how to do so properly.

What you need:

- 1 (20 ounces) can jackfruit, drained
- ¼ cup vegan ranch (recipe below)
- 10 ounces extra-firm tofu, drained and pressed dry

- ¾ cup water
- ¼ cup tapioca flour
- 2 teaspoons lemon juice
- ¾ teaspoon garlic powder
- 1 teaspoon salt
- ½ cup buffalo sauce
- ¼ cup vegan ranch (see recipe below)

What to do:

1. Drain the jackfruit and rinse thoroughly with cold water.
2. Transfer the pieces to a cutting board. Clean out the seeds.
3. Add the flesh of the jackfruit to a mixing bowl and pull apart by hand (there should be approximately 2 cups of flesh once done).
4. Blot with a paper towel to dry and set aside.
5. Ensure the tofu has been completely drained and pressed dry between a couple of sheets of paper towel.

6. There should be little moisture left when done.

7. Separate the tofu into pieces and add to a food processor.

8. Add in the water, tapioca flour, lemon juice, garlic powder, and salt.

9. Blend until completely smooth (do not add the jackfruit, as this will come later).

10. Preheat oven to 350 degrees Fahrenheit.

11. On medium to low heat, add the tofu mixture to a pan and allow to cook.

12. The mixture will begin to clump and become gooey after 4–5 minutes.

13. Once ready, add the jackfruit, buffalo sauce, and ranch, stirring to combine the ingredients together.

14. Remove from heat as soon as properly combined.

15. Pour the mixture into a prepared 9-inch cake tin or cast-iron skillet.

16. Bake until the top becomes golden brown

and the edges are bubbly (this takes approx. 15–20 minutes).

17. Remove the dip from the oven and stir, transferring to a small heated dish.

18. Serve hot with pita chips, celery, or sliced, toasted bread, or baguette.

Vegan Ranch 1

This vegan ranch sauce can be used with other dips and sauces or as is.

What you need:

- ½ cup extra-firm tofu, drained
- 1 teaspoon onion
- 1 teaspoon garlic powder
- ½ teaspoon black pepper
- ¼ teaspoon salt
- ¼ teaspoon dill
- 1 tablespoon dried parsley

- 1 tablespoon lemon juice

What to do:

1. Ensure the tofu has been completely drained and pressed dry between a couple of sheets of paper towel.

2. There should be little moisture left when done.

3. To make the ranch, combine together all the ingredients in a food processor and blend until completely smooth.

Calories: 103 kcal | Fat: 6 g | Carbohydrates: 5 g | Protein: 6 g

Vegan Ranch 2

This recipe is another way of making vegan ranch. It's tangier but just as delicious.

What you need:

- 1 cup vegan mayonnaise
- ½ teaspoon garlic
- ½ teaspoon onion powder

- ¼ teaspoon black pepper
- 2 teaspoons parsley, chopped
- 1 tablespoon dill, chopped
- ½ cup unsweetened soy milk (or nut milk of choice)

What to do:

1. Whisk everything together well.
2. Keep refrigerated.

Calories: 93 kcal | Fat: 9 g | Carbohydrates: 0 g | Protein: 0 g

BBQ Tahini

This recipe makes about 1 cup. Serving size is 2 tablespoons. You can do a lot with this sauce. Add more water to this sauce and turn it into a dressing to drizzle over salads. Spread it on bread for sandwiches. Add it to burgers and wraps. Use as a dip with raw veggies or chips.

What you need:

- 6 tablespoons tahini
- 3 tablespoons + 1 teaspoons tomato paste
- 2 teaspoons maple syrup
- ¾ teaspoon garlic powder
- 3 teaspoons apple cider vinegar
- 3 teaspoons molasses
- ¼ teaspoon liquid smoke
- Salt and pepper to taste
- ⅛ teaspoons chili powder (optional)
- ½ cup water (can use more or less depending on preferred consistency)

What to do:

1. Place all the ingredients, except the water, into a high-speed blender or food processor and blend until smooth.
2. Add in the water a bit at a time until the desired consistency is achieved.

Calories: 86 kcal

Vegan Sour Cream

Be sure to soak the cashews (either overnight or using hot water for at least 8 hours) before you begin.

This recipe makes 2 cups. Serving size is 2 tablespoons.

What you need:

- 1½ cups raw cashews
- ¾ cup water
- 2 tablespoons lemon juice
- 2 teaspoons apple cider vinegar
- ½ teaspoon sea salt

What to do:

1. Place cashews in a bowl and cover with water.
2. Soak overnight or for 8 hours using hot water.
3. Rinse and drain.
4. Place the drained cashews in a food processor.
5. Add the water, lemon, vinegar, and salt.
6. Blend on high until smooth, scraping down the

sides as you go.

7. Transfer into a small air-tight container and chill in the fridge.

8. You can freeze these in ice cube trays and use as needed. Set into a small bowl in the fridge to allow to defrost overnight.

Calories: 80 kcal | Fat: 6 g | Carbohydrates: 4 g | Protein: 3 g

Cheese Dip

What you need:

- 2 cups potatoes, mashed
- ¾ cup carrots, cubed and cooked
- ½ cup nutritional yeast flakes
- ⅓ cup extra virgin olive oil
- ⅓ cup water
- 1 tablespoon lemon juice
- 1 teaspoon salt

What to do:

1. Add your vegetables to a food processor.

2. Add in the nutritional yeast, oil, water, lemon juice, and salt.

3. Blend on high for 1–2 minutes until everything is smooth and creamy.

4. Serve hot over your favorite chips, as a dip for vegetables, or a spread for toasted sandwiches.

5. Store leftovers in an airtight container in the refrigerator.

6. Spice up the sauce to make a chunky dip by adding diced vegetables of your choice, such as jalapeños, green onions, tomatoes, black olives, or whatever else, and use as a topping for nachos.

Calories: 168 kcal | Carbohydrates: 12 g | Protein: 3 g | Fat: 12 g

Thai Peanut Sauce

This peanut sauce recipe is simple and easy and

requires no cooking. All you need to do is pop it in a pan, heat it up, and the sauce is done. It takes less than 15 minutes to make from start to finish.

What you need:

- ½ cup creamy peanut butter
- ¾ cup coconut milk
- 2 tablespoons red curry paste
- 2 tablespoons apple cider vinegar
- 2 tablespoons ground peanuts
- 1 tablespoon sugar (more or less to taste)
- Salt to taste

What to do:

1. Add your ingredients to a small bowl and whisk together well.
2. Transfer to a small saucepan. Bring to a boil. Whisk and remove from the heat.

Salad Dressing

Each salad needs a good drizzle of this amazing sauce. The key here is the nutritional yeast. It adds that tangy, cheesy flavor and gives the dressing body. Adding ¼ teaspoon of black pepper gives it a slight flavor without it tasting like pepper. Adding 1/2 teaspoon will give a peppery taste.

What you need:

- ⅔ cup raw pine nuts (you can substitute with cashews if you wish, but it will taste less authentic)
- ¼ cup + 3 tablespoons water
- 2 tablespoons lemon juice
- 2-3 tablespoons nutritional yeast flakes
- 2 large garlic cloves, crushed
- ½ teaspoon dried parsley
- ½ teaspoon ground pepper
- ½ teaspoon salt

What to do:

1. Add all of the ingredients to a high-powered blender or food processor and blend until smooth and creamy.

2. Pine nuts are softer than other nuts, so they should quickly blend smoothly.

3. If you have a weak blender and are using different nuts, I would suggest soaking the nuts overnight. Be sure to drain and rinse to prevent the texture from becoming gritty.

4. Refrigerate the sauce for 30 minutes before using. This dressing is perfect with any salad, and you could even drizzle a little over the lentil-tahini burgers for a summery taste.

Vegan Alfredo Sauce

Add this sauce to any pasta for a creamy, delicious meal. It is not recommended to substitute or eliminate any of these ingredients. The texture, taste, and consistency will be affected. Feel free to experiment though, if you wish. The lemon juice is also crucial as it eliminates the strong cashew flavor.

If you are using raw cashews and you do not have a high-powered blender, then you must soak them overnight in a bowl of water, drain, and rinse. It is better to use a food processor over a blender that is not very powerful. Rinsing the cashews will prevent it from becoming gritty instead of creamy.

What you need:

- 1½ cups white onion, diced
- 2 cups vegetable stock, divided
- ½ teaspoon salt
- ½ teaspoon black pepper
- 4 cloves garlic, minced
- ⅔ cups raw unsalted cashews
- 1–2 tablespoons lemon juice (start with just 1 and taste after blended, adjusting as needed)
- 2–4 tablespoons nutritional yeast

What to do:

1. Add onion and 1 cup of the stock to a large saucepan.

2. Turn up the heat to medium-high and cook approximately 8 minutes until the onion is very tender. Keep an eye on the onion to prevent burning. Turn down the heat as required.

3. Add the garlic and cook until fragrant. Be sure the stock has evaporated by now. If not, keep cooking until all the liquid has evaporated.

4. Too much liquid will reduce the thickness too much.

5. Add the cooked vegetables to a blender.

6. Add half the remaining stock and only add in more later as needed to adjust the consistency. You want it to be super thick and creamy, not too watery.

7. Add the remaining salt, pepper, yeast, and cashews. Blend until smooth.

8. Add in 1 tablespoon lemon juice. Taste it. Add more if desired.

9. Blend on high for a couple of minutes until very creamy and smooth.

10. Add more stock to adjust the consistency, as well as salt and pepper to taste.

11. Serve over preferred pasta. Note: When cooking your pasta, make sure to salt your water well. This will prevent the pasta from tasting bland and affecting the final taste of the dish.

Hummus

Hummus should not be thick and chunky. Dried chickpeas will result in a much better texture and flavor. Peel the chickpeas! The bean has a thin layer that you need to remove before mashing. As this recipe requires very few ingredients, try to use the highest quality possible. To make ice-cold water, simply place a few ice cubes in a glass of water for 5 minutes. The tahini should be smooth and runny.

What you need:

1. 2 cups dried chickpeas, soaked in water overnight

2. 1 teaspoon baking soda

3. 3–5 cloves garlic, crushed

4. 2 tablespoons lemon juice

5. 1½ teaspoons salt

6. ¼ cup tahini

7. 1 cup ice cold water, divided

What to do:

1. Soak the chickpeas in water for 12–24 hours, then drain and rinse them.

2. Add the chickpeas, garlic, and baking soda (the soda makes the chickpeas easier to peel) to an instant pot.

3. Cover with water until the level is 2 inches above the beans. Stir well and seal the cooker.

4. Cook on manual high pressure for 10–12 minutes. Let the pressure naturally release for 10 minutes *before* breaking the seal.

5. *If you do not have an instant pot or pressure cooker*: Add the chickpeas, garlic, and baking soda to a large pot and cover with water. Bring to a boil and cook for 40 minutes to 2 hours until the

beans are tender all the way through.

6. To peel the chickpeas, drain and rinse the cooked beans.

7. The skins will slide off quite easily when you gently "pinch" each bean. Discard the skins once finished.

8. To puree the chickpeas, add 3 cups, including the garlic, to a food processor.

9. In a separate bowl, combine the lemon juice and salt, stirring until the salt has dissolved. Set aside.

10. Turn the blender on, and pour the lemon juice into the mix while the machine is running.

11. Add the lemon juice slowly. Puree until smooth.

12. Add in the tahini. Seal the food processor and add ⅓ cup of water to the puree while the machine is running. Puree for 4–5 minutes. This will help make the hummus fluffy and smooth.

13. You can add in extra tahini and water in ¼

cup increments to adjust the consistency and fat content. (Note: Adding the cold water to the food processor while it is running is imperative if you want a light and fluffy result. The cool water reacts to the fat in the tahini, emulsifying it.)

14. Store in an airtight container for up to 5 days in the refrigerator. Serve with sliced vegetables of your choice, or use as a spread on burgers and sandwiches or as a dip for chips.

Walnut Butter

Use this as a spread for sandwiches or as an oil base while cooking or baking. This is a smoother, runnier kind of butter compared to almond or cashew butter. Walnut butter on its own is very nutty. Add in a pinch of salt, coconut sugar, or cocoa powder for flavor variations and to break the nutty flavor a bit.

What you need:

- 1½ cups raw, unsalted walnuts

What to do:

1. Preheat the oven to 300 degrees Fahrenheit.

2. Line a baking sheet with parchment paper.

3. Spread the walnuts on the pan in a thin layer.

4. Roast for 12 minutes until fragrant and a slight bit moist or oily on top.

5. Keep an eye on them so that they do not burn. They do not need to roast too long.

6. Add the roasted walnuts to a food processor and process for a 1 minute.

7. It should look like a chunky paste. Scrape down the sides and keep blending until it is smooth, oily, and runny.

Cashew Butter

Cashews are a much drier nut than the others due to the low oil content, so the result will be much drier and less runny than you would expect.

What you need:

- 2 cups raw, unsalted cashews (do not soak them as this will change the consistency and flavor too much)

What to do:

1. Add the raw cashews to a food processor.

2. They do not blend very well even in a high-powered blender, so a food processor is best.

3. Keep on whizzing until the cashew butter is soft and flowy, similar to cake frosting.

4. It takes up to 10 minutes to reach the right consistency.

5. Stop every 3 minutes or so, scraping down the sides as you go. (Note: Be patient and do not add any liquid.)

6. It will take several minutes, but just keep going until it gets to the paste stage.

7. Keep processing until it has a thick, creamy consistency, and then process even further until it is no longer stiff.

8. Before using in any recipe, ensure it has cooled off to room temperature.

9. Store in an airtight container in the pantry for up to 2 weeks or in the fridge for up to 2 months.

Calories: 100 kcal | Fat: 8.1 g | Protein: 2.7 g | Carbohydrates: 5.7 g

Roasted Almond Butter

Spread this over a toasted slice of bread of choice. Drizzle some maple syrup and a sprinkling of cinnamon for a sweet, delicious snack. Here are more ideas for using your almond butter:

1. with fruit or apple slices

2. to replace peanut butter on a sandwich

3. to replace oil in baking for desserts

You will definitely need a food processor for this recipe, as the nuts are hard to grind down without a bit of power.

What you need:

- 2 cups raw whole almonds

What to do:

1. Preheat an oven to 300 degrees Fahrenheit.

2. Prepare a baking sheet with parchment paper.

3. Place the almonds in a thin layer on the sheet.

4. Roast for 12–15 minutes until they start to smell really fragrant. Keep an eye on them so that they do not burn.

5. Remove from the oven and allow to cool slightly before adding them to a food processor.

6. Whizz the almonds for 5–10 minutes, scraping the sides as needed during the process.

7. You will need to do this a few times in the beginning to break up the clumps.

8. Keep whizzing, and do not add any liquid. It will not remain as a flour. Just keep on processing.

9. Do not stop too soon, or it will not become silky smooth. You want the consistency to be oily, dripping off the spoon.

Calories: 100 kcal | Fat: 8.1 g | Protein: 2.7 g | Carbohydrates: 5.7 g

Tomato-Basil Sauce

This is a gorgeous, fragrant sauce that is perfect with

pasta.

What you need:

- ¾ cup raw cashews, soaked and drained
- ¾ cup water
- 1 tablespoon lemon juice
- 2 cloves garlic, chopped
- ½ cup tomatoes, chopped
- ½ cup basil, chopped
- 2 tablespoons nutritional yeast

What to do:

1. In a blender or food processor, combine the cashews, water, lemon juice, garlic, tomatoes, basil, and nutritional yeast.
2. Whizz until smooth.
3. Scrape down the sides as needed, and keep whizzing until silky smooth.
4. Add to a small saucepan and bring to a boil.
5. Add a pinch of salt and pepper to taste.

6. Remove from heat and store in an airtight jar in the fridge.

Vegan Parmesan

What you need:

- ¾ cup raw cashews
- 3 tablespoons nutritional yeast
- ¾ teaspoon sea salt
- ¼ teaspoon garlic powder

What to do:

1. Do not soak the cashews beforehand. You want to keep the moisture to a minimum.
2. Add all your ingredients to the food processor.
3. Pulse until a fine meal is achieved. The cashews should be almost a rough floury texture.
4. Store in the refrigerator in an airtight container.

Chimichurri

If you are looking for an oil-free version, just substitute the same amount of aquafaba (the liquid in a can of chickpeas) for the olive oil.

This recipe makes 4 servings.

What you need:

- 1 cup fresh cilantro
- 1 cup parsley
- ¼ cup red onion, chopped
- ¼ cup olive oil
- 2 cloves garlic, minced
- 2 tablespoons lime juice
- ¼ teaspoon salt
- ¼ teaspoon red pepper flakes

What to do:

1. In a tall glass or bowl, add all the ingredients, and with an immersion blender, blend everything together.

2. If you prefer a textured sauce, you can stop as soon as everything has been just combined; otherwise, keep blending until the sauce is smooth.

Calories: 135 kcal (olive oil base), 9 kcal (aquafaba base)

Drinks

Strawberry Milk

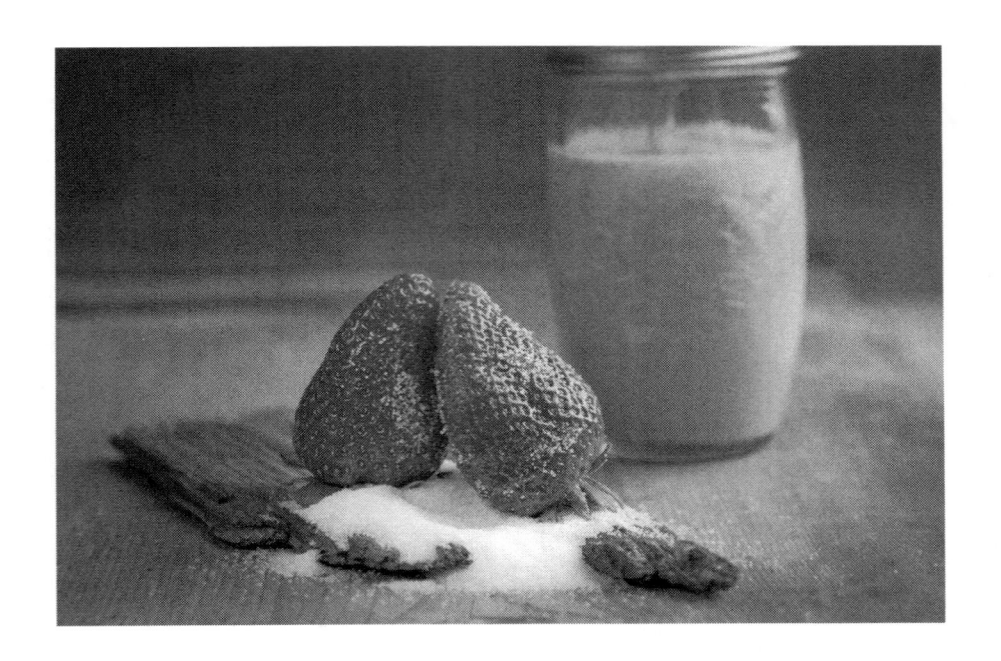

Even if strawberry milk isn't exactly your, well, cup of tea, you can still use this syrup over waffles or pancakes. Once you try this, you will surely be hooked. It tastes just like half-melted strawberry ice cream.

You can save the strawberry "mush" as a jam to be used in your oatmeal or spread on toast. You can even add it into the berry smoothie for breakfast or dessert! Other uses for this syrup:

1. Drizzle this sucker over pancakes.

2. Pour it onto waffles.

3. Stir it into porridge.

4. Pour it over French toast.

5. Mix it into hot chocolate.

6. Shake it into a cocktail.

To make strawberry milk, pour a glass of your favorite non-dairy milk and add the syrup to taste. Ta-da!

What you need:

- 2 cups strawberries, fresh preferred
- ½ cup water
- ¼ cup maple syrup (you can add more for a sweeter syrup)

What to do:

1. In a small cooking pot, add your ingredients and bring to a boil over medium-high heat.

2. Cook 10 minutes until the strawberries have turned incredibly soft.

3. Put a fine-mesh strainer over a bowl and pour the strawberry mixture through.

4. Using a spatula to squash the strawberries and liquid through as much as possible.

Calories: 25 kcal

You can substitute the strawberry syrup with pumpkin spice syrup. Make these syrups ahead of time and store in the fridge. While incredibly delicious, it is simply too much hassle to simmer spices and pumpkin with milk every time you want a pumpkin spice latte. To make a pumpkin spice latte or coffee, simply stir 1 tablespoon of syrup into your drink. You can adjust the amount to taste.

What you need:

- ¾ cup water
- ¾ cup brown sugar
- ¼ cup pumpkin, pureed
- 2 teaspoons pumpkin pie spice (see the recipe below if you want to make it yourself)

What to do:

1. In a small cooking pot, add your ingredients and bring to a boil over medium-high heat, whisking the ingredients together thoroughly.

2. Simmer approximately 3 minutes.

3. Pour the syrup through a fine-mesh strainer or a nut milk bag (allow to cool completely before using a nut milk bag).

4. To make a pumpkin spice latte or coffee, simply stir 1 tablespoon of syrup or into your latte or coffee to taste.

Calories: 56 kcal

For the pumpkin pie spice:

- 6 teaspoons cinnamon
- 1½ teaspoons ground ginger
- 1½ teaspoons nutmeg
- 1½ teaspoons allspice
- ¾ teaspoon ground cloves

Combine all the spices to a small, airtight jar. Shake until mixed well.

Calories: 12 kcal

Apple Cider

This recipe makes 8 servings. Make this, and your whole house will smell like heaven! It's delicious to share with your friends over the holidays.

What you need:

- 8 medium-sized apples (using softer apples will allow them to cook down faster, as well as keep you from tossing out the mushy ones)
- 2 medium-sized oranges
- 6 cinnamon sticks
- 1 teaspoon whole cloves
- 1 teaspoon allspice
- ½ cup dark-brown sugar
- 10 cups of water

What to do:

1. Wash and quarter the fruit. Keep the skins and

seeds.

2. Add the fruit to a large cooking pot and add in the remainder of the ingredients.
3. Bring to a boil and cook a few minutes before reducing to a simmer.
4. Allow to simmer for about 2 hours until the apples have broken down as much as possible.
5. Strain out the cooled liquid either through a fine-mesh strainer or a nut milk bag.
6. Discard the fruit pieces and serve hot with another cinnamon stick for garnish.

Calories: 140 kcal

Hot Christmas Rum

This recipe makes 2 servings.

You can add a large dollop of coconut cream on top and a sprinkle of cinnamon. While classic buttered rum has only water as a base, this one is meant to be slightly creamy. However, should you prefer the classic, simply substitute the milk and use a total of 1⅓ cups of water.

For an even creamier hot drink, substitute the water with more milk or some coconut cream.

What you need:

- 2 tablespoons brown sugar
- 1 tablespoon vegan butter
- 2 ounces of spiced rum (just enough for two servings)
- ⅛ teaspoon cinnamon
- ⅛ teaspoon nutmeg
- ⅔ cup almond milk (or dairy-free milk of your choice)
- ⅔ cup water

What to do:

1. Divide the rum between two mugs.
2. In a small pot on the stove, heat up the ingredients on low heat until the butter has melted completely. Whisk to incorporate the spices properly.
3. Allow it to simmer for 2 minutes before pouring

into the mugs.

4. You can also divide the ingredients evenly between the two mugs, and heat the milk in the microwave.

Calories: 215 kcal

Chapter 6: The Plant-Based Meal Plan

While following this meal plan, you should listen to what your body needs. This has been tailored to accommodate the caloric needs of an average female who needs approximately 1,700 calories a day in order to maintain current weight. However, if you feel weak and without energy, add in an extra light meal, adjusting as needed. Starting with smaller portions will be more effective in hitting the perfect spot without the risk of overeating.

Should you adjust the meal plan to be able to lose weight, do not reduce the intake of calories by more than 300 calories per day as this could negatively affect your health, especially if the reduction will put you below your BMR. (Again, the estimation is guided by the 1,700 caloric requirements of a slightly active or sedentary person.)

Most breakfasts are light; however, you can switch out the menu as you see fit. Keep in mind, though, that not all recipes are equal in caloric values. So if you need, for example, more protein, add a meal that is higher in protein.

Additionally, should you be combining this with a complementary dietary protocol, such as intermittent fasting, you can adjust the plan as needed.

Note: Breakfast is simply marked as such due to the nature of it being the first meal of the day. This does not mean you have to eat it when you wake up, and you can push it back to when you get to work, school, or whenever it is most convenient. Just do not skip meals.

You will notice that there have been no desserts added to the menu although they do appear in the recipe lists. This is due to the fact that while these are plant-based and vegan-friendly, too much of a good thing is not necessarily healthy. These items still contain some form of sugar, an ingredient that still needs to be limited regardless of preferred foods.

However, do not be scared to add in a small scoop of ice cream or a slice of cheesecake to round out your meals for the day. (Just remember to stay within your body's required caloric range.)

Week 1

1. Monday

    - Breakfast: mocha smoothie and chickpea and onion omelet
    - Lunch: sloppy joe
    - Dinner: spicy squash soup and a slice of zucchini bread

2. Tuesday

    - Breakfast: gingerbread waffles with a generous scoop of nut butter of choice and fruits of choice
    - Lunch: crispy tofu stir-fry
    - Dinner: tomato soup

3. Wednesday

    - Breakfast: blueberry smoothie and crepes
    - Lunch: avo-kale-veggie bowl
    - Dinner: mac and cheese

4. Thursday

- Breakfast: tofu scramble and toasted zucchini bread
- Lunch: mushroom soup
- Dinner: chili and grilled butternut side

5. Friday
    - Breakfast: pumpkin cookies and cinnamon smoothie
    - Lunch: orange-tofu stir-fry
    - Dinner: mushroom burger and summer salad

6. Saturday
    - Breakfast: peanut butter smoothie and vegan French toast
    - Lunch: lentil-tahini burger and summer salad
    - Dinner: chickpea meatball and romaine salad

7. Sunday
    - Breakfast: berry smoothie and pancakes
    - Lunch: mushroom and zucchini bowl
    - Dinner: cashew stew and roasted vegetable side

Week 2

8. Monday

    - Breakfast: pancakes
    - Lunch: cauli-korma
    - Dinner: zucchini lasagna (double serving) and summer salad side

9. Tuesday

    - Breakfast: mocha smoothie and toasted cinnamon-apple bread
    - Lunch: choc chip granola and pancakes
    - Dinner: crispy tofu stir-fry

10. Wednesday

    - Breakfast: mint choc-chip smoothie
    - Lunch: lunchbox sandwich and crispy tofu salad
    - Dinner: mac and cheese (double serving)

11. Thursday

    - Breakfast: blueberry smoothie and pancakes

- Lunch: tortilla roll-ups and roasted vegetables side
- Dinner: Avo-kale-veggie bowl

12. Friday
    - Breakfast: tofu scramble
    - Lunch: tomato soup and zucchini bread
    - Dinner: veggie Bolognese

13. Saturday
    - Breakfast: pumpkin cookies and breakfast grits bowl
    - Lunch: mushroom soup and zucchini bread
    - Dinner: sweet potato curry

14. Sunday
    - Breakfast: peanut butter smoothie and pancakes
    - Lunch: Noodle soup
    - Dinner: Orange-tofu stir-fry with roasted cauli-wedges and roasted summer veggies

Week 3

15. Monday

- Breakfast: sun-dried tomato quiche and a slice of zucchini bread
- Lunch: chili
- Dinner: lentil-tahini burger and roasted butternut side

16. Tuesday

- Breakfast: pancakes
- Lunch: avo-and-noodle salad
- Dinner: black bean and mushroom burger with spring salad

17. Wednesday

- Breakfast: tomato soup and zucchini bread
- Lunch: spring salad and sun-dried tomato quiche
- Dinner: mushroom and zucchini bowl

18. Thursday

- Breakfast: cinnamon-apple bread with nut butter of choice and fresh fruit
- Lunch: black bean burger and summer salad
- Dinner: veggie meatloaf

19. Friday

    - Breakfast: chickpea and onion omelet
    - Lunch: sloppy joe and spring salad
    - Dinner: butternut and cashew stew

20. Saturday

    - Breakfast: tortilla roll-ups and breakfast grits bowl
    - Lunch: mac and cheese
    - Dinner: cauli-korma

21. Sunday

    - Breakfast: vegan French toast (double serving)
    - Lunch: mushroom and asparagus bowl
    - Dinner: black bean tostada

Week 4

22. Monday

- Breakfast: creamy orange smoothie and crepes with fruits of choice
- Lunch: veggie Bolognese
- Dinner: zucchini lasagna

23. Tuesday

- Breakfast: pumpkin cookies and chickpea and onion omelet
- Lunch: sweet potato curry
- Dinner: lentil-tahini burger

24. Wednesday

- Breakfast: blueberry smoothie and gingerbread waffles
- Lunch: orange-tofu stir-fry

- Dinner: crispy tofu salad

25. Thursday

    - Breakfast: spicy squash soup

    - Lunch: lentil-tahini burger

    - Dinner: mac and cheese (double serving)

26. Friday

    - Breakfast: avo-and-noodle salad

    - Lunch: chickpea and black bean burger

    - Dinner: avo-kale-veggie bowl

27. Saturday

    - Breakfast: fig and arugula salad

    - Lunch: mushroom and zucchini bowl with two slices zucchini bread

    - Dinner: mushroom soup

28. Sunday

    - Breakfast: mocha smoothie and fig and arugula salad

- Lunch: butternut and chickpea stew

- Dinner: tomato soup

Conclusion

Incorporating more vegetables into your diet will certainly improve your health and energy levels. Moreover, the sheer variety and combinations you can work with are both fun and satisfying. Feel free to experiment with different types of vegetables to create more dishes you will fall in love with.

Do not forget to grab a couple of cookies and a scoop of ice cream from the dessert menu to help curb that sweet-tooth craving. Just do not overdo it.

Should you experience any adverse effects, please consult your general practitioner. This book is not meant to be used to replace the advice of licensed medical practitioners. Listen to what your body needs and adjust accordingly.

Hungry? Eat a slightly larger serving. Do not starve yourself, and soon you will reap the benefits of following a delicious plant-based diet.

Ask your family and friends to enjoy these hearty, delicious meals with you, making this diet a festive family affair.

Printed in Great Britain
by Amazon